GERIATRIC PSYCHOPHARMACOLOGY

DEVELOPMENTS IN NEUROLOGY

GERIATRIC PSYCHOPHARMACOLOGY

KALIDAS NANDY, Editor
*Geriatric Research, Education and Clinical Center, Veterans Administration
Medical Center, Bedford, Massachusetts, and Department of Anatomy and
Neurology, Boston University School of Medicine, Boston, Massachusetts,
U.S.A.*

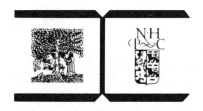

ELSEVIER/NORTH-HOLLAND
NEW YORK · AMSTERDAM · OXFORD

© 1979 by Elsevier North Holland, Inc.

with the exception of those articles lacking a copyright line on their opening
chapter pages whose copyrights reside with the individual authors and those
articles written by United States Government employees which are works of the
United States Government and cannot be copyrighted.

Published by:

Elsevier North Holland, Inc.
52 Vanderbilt Avenue, New York, New York 10017

Sole distributors outside U.S.A. and Canada:

Elsevier/North-Holland Biomedical Press
335 Jan van Galenstraat, P.O. Box 211
Amsterdam, The Netherlands

Library of Congress Cataloging in Publication Data

Main entry under title:

Geriatric psychopharmacology.
    (Developments in neurology ; v. 3)

    Bibliography: p.
    Includes index.
    1. Geriatric pharmacology.   2. Psychopharmacology.   I. Nandy, Kalidas.
    II. Series.   [DNLM: 1. Psychopharmacology—In old age—Congresses.
    W1 DE998E v. 3 / QV77 G369 1979]
RC953.7.G47   615'.78   79-9168
ISBN: 0-444-80078-6 (series)
ISBN: 0-444-00339-8 (volume)

Manufactured in the United States of America

Contents

Preface

With the current trend of the population growth resulting from significant extension of the median lifespan all over the world, particularly in the developed countries, the number of older people had a dramatic increase in the past decades. According to the U. S. Census Bureau there are over 21 million Americans 65 years and older at the present time. It has been projected that there might be 40 million people over 65 years and 16 million people over 75 years by the turn of the century. Current hospital and nursing home statistics indicate that 10 percent of the 65 and older group, 25 percent of the 75 and older group and 50 percent of 90 years and older group suffer from a significant degree of mental impairment. If this trend continues, senile dementia could amount to a very serious problem of the health care system in the United States. It is expected that 1 out of 3 American males will be Veterans by the year 1990. The Veterans Administration being a large component of the health care system is also faced with the serious problem of providing care to large numbers of older veterans with many age-related diseases including severe mental impairment.

The success of the treatment of these cases with mental impairment in geriatric population will not only depend on the early diagnosis of the disease process but also on a thorough understanding of the various drug therapies. It is, therefore, important that physicians are not only cognigent of the proper applications of the various pharmaco-therapeutic agents but also have an understanding of the underlying pharmacokinetics and drug interactions. This book will deal with the subject in three sections. The first section will deal primarily with mode of action of drugs and pharmacokinetics. The second section will be devoted to evaluation of the patients and proper drug therapy including indications and contraindications. The third section will contain detailed discussion of the rather newer groups of psychoactive

drugs which might appear promising in this field. It is hoped that this book
will be helpful to the physicians and different specialties as well as
scientists involved in investigation research in geriatric medicine.

The editor is grateful to James C. Crutcher, M.D., Chief Medical Director,
Veterans Administration Central Office, for permission to edit the book. I
am also indebted to Paul A. L. Haber, M.D., Assistant Chief Medical Director
for Professional Services, Ralph Goldman, M.D., Assistant Chief Medical
Director for Extended Care, Francis A. Zacharewicz, M.D., Medical Director,
Ms. Dorothy Sassenrath, M.S., Educational Specialist, South Central Regional
Medical Education Center, Veterans Administration.

Finally, the editor expresses his sincere thanks to the publisher for the
continued cooperation and understanding in dealing with the problems in the
preparation of this volume.

K. NANDY

Foreword

It is a signal honor for me to be asked to contribute the foreword to this text on Geriatric Psychopharmacology. Dr. Kalidas Nandy has been active in this field for much of his professional career and has assembled a group of papers as much distinguished for their scholarliness as their empathy for the solution to the problem of mental derangement in the elderly.

It has been estimated that three quarters of the mental disturbances in the elderly could be favorably affected if knowledge already in hand could be successfully applied to those problems. That is to say, that no new knowledge is required for the successful intervention in the management problems of millions of elderly patients now suffering from some form of mental perturbation. The sad fact is, that scanty knowledge, indifferently applied only serves to increase the misery of patients with mental problems.

The emergence of the science of psychopharmacology has created a revolution in the treatment of mental disorders. It has resulted in the disappearance of large, back-ward warehouses for the incarceration of psychiatric patients. Just so, the long-term care of elderly patients with psychiatric problems could be vastly improved by skillful application of current psychopharmaceutical technology.

The emergence of new detailed knowledge of the production, metabolic fate and dispersion of the biogenic amines has only made the potential of geriatric psychopharmacology more immediate. If we are to prevent the pharmacologic straightjacket of the past, and if we are to explore new possibilities of favorably intervening in the mental distress of the aging, this text will help mark the way.

PAUL A.L. HABER, M.D.

Contributors

PAUL T. CARROL, Ph.D., Assistant Professor, Department of Pharmacology and Toxicology, University of Rhode Island, Kingston, Rhode Island.

STANLEY CATH, M.D., Medical Director, Family Advisory Service and Treatment Center, Inc., 18 Moore Street, Belmont, Massachusetts.

JONATHAN O. COLE, M.D., Chief, Psychopharmacology Program, McLean Hospital, Belmont, Massachusetts and Consultant, Boston State Hospital, Boston, Massachusetts.

ALBERT FANCHAMPS, M.D., Medical Counsel, Pharmaceutical Research and Development, Sandoz Ltd., Basel, Switzerland.

CHARLES M. GAITZ, M.D., Head, Department of Applied Research, Texas Research Institute of Mental Sciences, Houston, Texas.

RALPH GOLDMAN, M.D., Assistant Chief Medical Director for Extended Care, V.A. Central Office, Washington, D. C.

PAUL A. L. HABER, M.D., Assistant Chief Medical Director for Professional Services, V. A. Central Office, Washington, D.C.

JAMES T. HARTFORD, M.D., Texas Research Institute of Mental Sciences, Houston, Texas.

SIEGFRIED HOYER, M.D., Professor, Department of Pathochemistry and General Neurochemistry, University of Heidelberg, D-6900 Heidelberg, Germany.

ZAFAR H. ISRAILI, Ph.D., Professor of Chemistry and Associate Professor of Medicine, Emory University School of Medicine, Atlanta, Georgia.

A. L. JATON, Preclinical Research, Pharmaceutical Division, Sandoz, Ltd., Basel, Switzerland.

BESSEL VAN DER KOLK, M.D., Chief, Psychopharmacology, V. A. Outpatient Clinic, and Associate Clinical Professor of Psychiatry, Tufts Medical School, Boston, Massachusetts.

AMOS D. KORCZYN, M.D., M.Sc., Visiting Associate Professor, Department of Neurology, Mount Sinai Hospital, New York, and Associate Professor of Neuropharmacology, Tel Aviv.

MILTON KRAMER, M.D., Director, Dream-Sleep Laboratory, Veterans Administration Hospital, and Professor of Psychiatry, University of Cincinnati, Cincinnati, Ohio.

HARBANS LAL, Ph.D., Professor of Pharmacology and Toxicology, University of Rhode Island, Kingston, Rhode Island.

DIETER M. LOEW, M.D., Preclinical Research, Pharmaceutical Division, Sandoz Ltd., Basel, Switzerland.

MICHAEL J. MALONE, M.D., Director, Geriatric Research, Education and Clinical Center, V. A. Hospital, Bedford, Massachusetts and Professor of Neurology and Psychiatry, Boston University School of Medicine, Boston, Massachusetts.

KALIDAS NANDY, M.D., Ph.D., Associate Director, Geriatric Research, Education and Clinical Center, V. A. Hospital, Bedford, Massachusetts, and Professor of Anatomy and Neurology, Boston University School of Medicine, Boston, Massachusetts.

KENNETH NOBEL, M.D., Instructor, Department of Psychiatry, Harvard Medical School, Boston, Massachusetts.

DONALD S. ROBINSON, M.D., Professor and Chairman of Pharmacology and Professor of Medicine, Marshall University School of Medicine, Huntington, West Virginia.

CARL SALZMAN, M.D., Associate Professor of Psychiatry, Harvard Medical School, Boston, Massachusetts.

J. M. VIGOURET, Preclinical Research, Pharmaceutical Division, Sandoz Ltd., Basel, Switzerland.

HSIOH-SHAN WANG, M.D., Professor of Psychiatry, Duke University Medical

Center, Durham, North Carolina.
MELVIN D. YAHR, M.D., Professor and Chairman, Department of Neurology,
  Mount Sinai School of Medicine, New York, New York.
WILLIAM W. K. ZUNG, M.D., Professor of Psychiatry, Duke University
  Medical Center, Durham, North Carolina.

RALPH GOLDMAN, M. D.
Assistant Chief Medical Director for Extended Care,
VA Central Office, Washington, D.C.   20420

INTRODUCTION

It has become trite to remind readers that the population is aging. It
is more important that although there is a growing body of basic data defining a variety of changes resulting from aging, most physicians still do
not have an integrated concept of the aging process, apart from the overt,
external pattern seen in the individuals around us. As a result, there is
little knowledge of or instruction on treatment modifications which are
appropriate to different ages. Most physicians must rely on experience
alone. Texts which present documented authority to support modes of treatment which adjust for age and the infirmities of age are only now beginning
to appear.

As he has done several times before, Dr. Nandy has brought together an
outstanding panel of experts who explore one aspect of geriatric pharmacology, the management of psychiatric impairment. There is an obvious need
for state-of-the art presentations in this area of concern. With the rapid
development to be expected, it is necessary to establish perspectives which
can be kept current by practice, ongoing education, and the periodic re-pre-
sentation of similar, overview material.

Depression and intellectual deterioration are two of the most prevalent
conditions facing the geriatric practitioner. They are a tragic burden to
the patients, difficult to treat, and demoralizing to the family and society.
The resultant loss of ability to relate and interact socially alienates
family and friends, and is a major factor leading to institutionalization.
Any techniques that delay or ameliorate these problems will be major
triumphs. I believe that this volume will mark a significant achievement
in the pursuit of these goals.

I
Pharmacokinetics

Published 1979 by Elsevier North Holland, Inc.
Nandy, Ed. Geriatric Psychopharmacology

ALTERATIONS IN BRAIN NEUROTRANSMITTER

SYSTEMS RELATED TO SENESCENCE

HARBANS LAL AND PAUL T. CARROLL
  Department of Pharmacology & Toxicology
University of Rhode Island, Kingston, RI   02881

INTRODUCTION

   The CNS is organized to perform its functions through neuronal intercommuni-
cations that are accomplished at billions of synapses. Many CNS functions become slow and less efficient in the senescent subjects. Particularly, transmission over multisynaptic pathways is substantially reduced. The transmission
at a synapse is intimately related to the functioning of specific neurotransmitters.

   A neurotransmitter is released from the pre-synaptic sites as a result of
pre-synaptic neuronal activity. This transmitter then diffuses in the synaptic
gap to the sites where specific receptors for this neurotransmitter are located.
There the transmitter is attracted by the receptors to which it binds. The receptors are structurally specialized spots on the neuronal membrane which have
a high affinity for specific neurotransmitters and contain a transduction mechanism that allows the neurotransmitter, once bound, to translate its interaction
into a biochem sequellae that lead ultimately to the observed response. The nature of the transducing mechanisms remains a "black box," but a critical role
of "second messengers" have been well recognized.

   Cyclic neucleotides have been proposed to act as "second messengers" in a
number of neurotransmitter controlled synaptic actions in the CNS. In order to
accomplish the specific actions synapse specific neucleotides (cyclic AMP and
cyclic GMP) are produced by the action of neurotransmitters on a class of enzymes called nucleotide cyclases.

   Over the past 25 years, progressive analyses of the synthesis, storage, release, conservation, catabolism and the actions of brain neurotransmitters as
well as activity of nucleotide cyclases and associated protein kinases have
suggested that the neurotransmitters are involved in many brain functions,
mental disease states and bases for pharmacological intervention in a variety
of conditions. However, research on the changes in the neurotransmitter functions that occur in the senescence related brain dysfunctions is, at best, in
its infancy as a scientific discipline. Most experiments are limited to exploration of a small segment of this area. The important problem of defining

the senescence in animals or obtaining human material free of diseases is difficult to solve. Species and strain differences are marked. Animal models are difficult to establish. This review is an early attempt to summarize a number of studies completed to date and present an integrated view of brain neurotransmitter dysfunctions that are associated with senescence. No attempt was made to present comprehensive literature review.

CHOLINERGIC SYSTEM.

Acetylcholine (ACh) is an established neurotransmitter substance in the brain. ACh is synthesized from acetate and choline by the enzyme, choline-o-acetyltransferase (ChAT). ACh is present in the cytoplasm as well as vesicles of the nerve ending. It is released into the synaptic cleft where it acts on ACh specific receptors to produce a "second messenger" substance and is subsequently hydrolyzed by the enzyme, acetylcholinesterase (AChE). The degradation product choline is recycled for ACh synthesis inside cholinergic neurons following its uptake.

Because of a lack of well accepted histochemical technique to localize cholinergic pathways in the brain, precise distribution of all cholinergic neurons in the CNS is not known. However, based upon combined anatomical and biochemical approaches a number of cholinergic systems have been identified. The septo-hippocampal system is the most widely recognized. The caudate nucleus contains cholinergic neurons terminating within the nucleus. Cholinergic neurons originating from the centro median nucleus in the thalamus also terminate in the caudate. A habenulointerpeduncular cholinergic track has also been recognized.

Precise functions for brain cholinergic systems remains undefined. However, their involvement in learning, memory, motor and affective functions have been widely postulated. They also seem to be exerting controls on endocrine functions.

Neurological manifestations of aging in most animal species include progressive loss of memory and deterioration in learning.[1-3] The role of the neurotransmitter ACh in learning and memory is well documented[4-10] and consequently one might predict that some aspect of central ACh metabolism might be impaired in senescent animals. Several groups of investigators have reported alterations in various parameters of central ACh metabolism in the aged brains of the following animal species: rats[11-18], mice[19-22], monkeys[24], and humans.[25]

Those parameters of central ACh metabolism that have been studied in the aged animal include the activity of the two enzymes, choline-o-acetyltransferase and acetylcholinesterase, the levels of ACh, choline transport, and the calcum dependent, potassium induced release of ACh from brain synaptosomes.

Generally, most investigators have reported that the activity of both ChAT[25,23,18,21] and AChE[16,11,15,16,24] are reduced in some brain regions of senescent mice and rats.

Although the brain levels of ACh in aged animals do not differ from those of adult animals,[17-18] the brain levels of ACh in young and old animals are significantly reduced by administration of d-amphetamine whereas the brain level of ACh in the adult animals is unaffected.[17] This result may suggest that ACh turnover in the brains of young and old animals may be differentially sensitive to drugs as compared with adult animals.

The transport of the ACh precursor, choline, into brain tissue occurs by high and low affinity processes:[26,27-28] the high affinity process is believed to be rate limiting in ACh synthesis[26,29-30] and might thereby be very sensitive to the aging process. Additionally, extracellular choline which is transported into brain tissue is utilized for the potassium induced release of ACh.[31-33] Recently one group of investigators reported that the "high affinity" choline transport process into synaptosomes prepared from the aged mouse (12 months) is significantly reduced relative to the young mouse.[22] This same group was unable to detect an impairment in the secretory process of ACh release in the brains of old mice. Both high and low affinity choline transport processes in forebrain minces of senescent mice (14 months) appear to be reduced to the same extent (30%) with a comparable decrease in ACh formed relative to 4 month control mice (P.T. Carroll, unpublished observations). Thus further work is required to determine whether choline transport into cholinergic nerve endings of brain tissue is specifically impaired during senescence and whether this parameter of central ACh metabolism is the most sensitive to the aging process.

Availability of high specific activity H^3 quinuclidinyl benzilate (QNB) with specific binding affinity to cholinergic muscarinic receptors in the brain has stimulated a number of studies to obtain information on the cholinergic receptors in the senescent subjects. Usually these receptors have been found to be unaffected. However, in Alzheimer's disease, QNB binding is markedly reduced in hippocampus[34] with a trend in reduction in substantia nigra and amygdala[35] and no change in cortex, caudate, nucleus accumbens, thalamus, midbrain or pons. The saturation studies in the hippocampus indicated that the changes in QNB binding was not due to affinity changes.[34]

There are reports that the pharmacological responsivity of cholinergic systems is increased in the senescence.[16,36] The old animals require smaller

TABLE 1

MAJOR CATECHOLAMINERGIC SYSTEMS[1]

System	Origin	Site(s) of Termination
D O P A M I N E R G I C S Y S T E M S		
Meso-telencephalic[2] Nigrostriatal	Substantia nigra, pars compacta; ventral tegmental area	Neostriatum (caudate-putamen), globus pallidus
Mesocortical	Ventral tegmental area; substantia nigra, pars compacta	Isocortex (mesial frontal, anterior cingulate, entorhinal, perirhinal) Allocortex (olfactory bulb, anterior olfactory nucleus, olfactory tubercle, piriform cortex, septal area, nucleus accumbens, amygdaloid complex)
Tubero-hypophysial	Arcuate and periventricular hypothalamic nuclei	Neuro-intermediate lobe of pituitary, median eminence
Retinal	Interplexiform cells, of retina	Inner and outer plexiform layers of retina
Incerto-hypothalamic	Zona incerta, posterior hypothalamus	Dorsal hypothalamic area, septum
Periventricular	Medulla in area of dorsal motor vagus, nucleus tractus solitarius, periaqueductal and periventricular gray	Periventricular and periaqueductal gray, tegmentum, tectum, thalamus, hypothalamus
Olfactory bulb	Periglomerular cells	Glomeruli (mitral cells)
N O R A D R E N E R G I C S Y S T E M S[3]		
Locus coeruleus	Locus coeruleus	Spinal cord, brainstem, cerebellum, hypothalamus, thalamus, basal telencephalon, and the entire isocortex
Lateral tegmental	Dorsal motor vagus, nucleus tractus solitarius, and adjacent tegmentum, lateral tegmentum	Spinal cord, brainstem, hypothalamus, basal telencephalon
A D R E N E R G I C S Y S T E M S		
Dorsal tegmental and lateral tegmental	Caudal medulla	Spinal cord, brainstem (locus coeruleus, periaqueductal gray), hypothalamus, thalamus

[1] Adopted from Moore and Bloom (1978, 1979).
[2] The term meso-telencephalic refers to the projections of the midbrain dopamine neurons upon the telencephalon. See text for description.
[3] The brainstem norepinephrine neurons located in the dorsal, caudal, medulla medially and laterally are considered, along with the pontine and isthmic cell groups, to constitute one system.

doses of atropine to block ACh effects on the rabbit heart, less of a curare-like agent to block neuromuscular transmission in the rat, less ganglionic stimulant to contract the nictitating membrane of the cat or slow the heart rate of vagotomized rats. Old rats and cats also require greater voltages of stimulation of the vagus nerve to produce tachy cardia. The threshold dose of ACh given into the cerebral ventricle to produce EEG, cardiovascular, and respiratory changes is smaller in the aged animals. The most pronounced difference in ACh response occurs in the sensorimotor cortex, hippocampus, and amygdala and the least in the medulla oblongata, reticularis portis, and piriform cortex. The locomotor activity as stimulated by anticholinergic drugs or depressed by cholinergic stimulant is markedly altered in the senescent mice.[36]

CATECHOLAMINERGIC SYSTEMS

The CNS contains at least three types of catecholamines (CA): dopamine (DA), norepinephrine (NE) and epinephrine (E). A summary of the organization of the major CA systems is given in Table 1.

DA neuronal systems are principally located in the upper mesencephalon and dicephalon. They vary anatomically from systems of neurons without axons (retina, olfactory bulb) and with very restricted projections, to systems with extensive axonal arborizations. In contrast to NE systems, the DA systems appear to be "local" systems with highly specified and topographically organized projections. The efferent trajectories of NE systems are more widespread with a high degree of collateral arborization and marked propensity for the expression of post-lesion regrowth. Existence of separate and distinctive E systems have been realized only recently and not enough is known to characterize their anatomical and physiological characteristics.

It has been known for many years that in the age-related disease of Parkinsonism there is significant loss of dopaminergic neurons. However, in recent years, a similar loss has been reported in normal subjects of advanced age.[15,25,37] The alterations in CA systems are extensive. The available data are summarized in Table 2-3. Although data vary from one researcher to another, several conclusions can be made based upon the trends.

The idea that catecholamine synthesis and turnover is reduced in senescent subjects is suggested by the finding that tyrosine hydroxylase, the enzyme believed to be rate limiting in CA synthesis, is found to be deficient in activity in these subjects. This decrease in CA synthesis is found in many areas of the brain and is not related to any deficit in the availability or uptake of catecholamine precursors.[41]

TABLE 2

EFFECT OF SENESCENCE ON BRAIN ENZYMES RELATED TO CATECHOLAMINE SYSTEMS

Test Subjects	Brain Area	Age of Comparison	Change	Reference
T Y R O S I N E H Y D R O X Y L A S E				
Human	Amygdala	20 vs 50 y	−61%	37
"	Putamen	"	−48%	"
"	Caudate	"	−39%	"
"	Globus Pallidus	"	−33%	"
"	N. accumbens	"	−31%	"
"	Substantia nigra	15 vs 60 y	−50%	40
"	Hypothalamus	"	0%	"
Rat	Neostriatum	4-15 vs 25-28 m	−35%	15
"	Brain minus cerebbelum and neostriatum	"	0%	15
D O P A D E C A R B O X Y L A S E				
Human	Amygdala	20 vs 50 y	−72%	37
"	Putamen	"	−54%	"
"	Caudate	"	−35%	"
"	Globus Pallidus	"	35-55%	"
"	N. accumbens	"	−47%	"
"	Septal area	"	−27%	"
"	Substantia nigra	"	−49%	"
Mouse	Neostriatum	12 vs 28 m	0%	41
"	Hypothalamus	"	0%	41
C A T E C H O L - O - M E T H Y L T R A N S F E R A S E				
Human	Caudate	70 vs 90 yrs	decrease	42
"	Putamen	"	0	42
"	Frontal Cortex	"	increase	42
M O N O A M I N E O X I D A S E				
Human	Hindbrain	25-55 vs 65 y	+50%	43,44
"	Globus Pallidus	45 vs 45 y	increase	45
"	Thalamus	"	"	"
"	Hypothalamus	"	"	"
"	Hippocampus	"	"	"
"	Substantia nigra	"	"	"
"	Reticular Activating System	"	"	"
"	Cortex	"	"	"
"	Caudate nucleus	"	"	"

TABLE 3

EFFECT OF SENESCENCE ON BRAIN CATECHOLAMINE LEVELS

Test Subjects	Brain Area	Age of Comparison	Change	Reference
		D O P A M I N E		
Human	Caudate	73 vs 73 y	decrease	46
"	Globus Pallidus	"	"	"
"	Putamen	"	"	"
"	Hypothalamus	"	0	"
"	Red. nucleus	"	0	"
"	Substantia nigra	"	0	"
Mouse	Whole brain	12 vs 28 m	0	41
"	" "	10-12 vs 28-30 m	0	41
"	Neostriatum	12 vs 28 m	- 20%	41
"	"	10-12 vs 28-30 m	- 30%	41
Rat	Brain (-neostriatum and cerebellum)	7 vs 24-29 m	0	15
		N O R E P I N E P H R I N E		
Human	Hindbrain	25 vs 65+y	- 40%	44
"	Hypothalamus	73 vs 73 y	decrease	46
"	Pineal gland	y vs old	0	47
Mouse	Whole brain	12 vs 28 m	0	41
"	" "	9 vs 28 m	0	48
"	Cerebellum	12 vs 28 m	0	41
"	Hypothalamus	"	0	41
"	Brainstem	"	0	41
Monkey	Brainstem	6 vs 10 y	decrease	42
"	Hypothalamus	"	decrease	42
Rat	Whole brain (-neostriatum and cerebellum	7 vs 24-28 m	0	15
Chick	Hemispheres	10 vs 36	0	49
"	Cerebellum	"	0	49
		H O M O V A N I L L I C A C I D		
Human	Cerebrospinal fluid	30 vs 80 y	+50%	50

In addition, there is a marked decrease in the levels of dopamine in the
striatum; no change in norepinephrine levels is noted in this area. These findings suggest that either the synthetic apparatus of neurons is damaged or that
a significant number of neurons containing this apparatus have been degenerated
in the senescent subjects. Upon careful examination both deficits are found
to occur. There is a marked decline in the synthetic enzymes as well as a significant decrease in the dopaminergic cell population in aged subjects. These
deficits are present both in experimental animals as well as in elderly human
subjects.

Other enzymes involved in CA synthesis and metabolism such as DOPA decarboxylase, catechol-0-methyl transferase (COMT), and monoamine oxidase, are
also altered in senescence. Although, both tyrosine hydroxylase and DOPA
decarboxylase are altered to a much greater extent than the changes in ChAT
and GAD. Monoamine oxidase, responsible for oxidative deamination of brain
amines both in cytoplasm and extracellularly, tends to increase during aging.
This change is limited to neuronal tissue, as monoamine oxidase in the liver
is not altered with senescence. The only nonneuronal tissue in which monoamine oxidase is increased is the plasma platelet. Brain COMT does not show
a consistent trend in the mouse or monkey. However, there is marked decrease
in COMT in human caudate with senescence.

No significant change in the serotonin system in relation to senescence
has been reported. The studies focusing on this system are summarized in
Table 4.

Very little is known about the changes in cyclic nucleotides in senescent
subjects. A significant decrease in the levels of cyclic AMP in the cerebral
cortex of aged rats was reported by Zimmerman and Berg.[51] However, Puri and
Volicer[52] could not confirm that finding. Similarly, Makman (personal communication) could not find any adenylate cyclase change in the rabbit brain. However, there develops a marked reduction in the sensitivity of striatal
adenylate cyclase to dopamine both in the rat (Figure 1) and in the rabbit.
The data summarized in Figure 1 indicate that dopamine induced stimulation
of adenylate cyclase declines gradually with advancing age in the rat.
Rats of 24 or 30 months of age show little responsivity to any concentration
of dopamine with respect to striatal adenylate cyclase stimulation. Similar
reduction in the sensitivity to dopamine has also been confirmed in the
rabbit. Makman also showed that the adenylate cyclase sensitivity to NE,
isoproterenol and histamine was also reduced in the aged rabbits. The sensitivity of the same adenylate cyclase to fluoride was not altered.[52]

TABLE 4

EFFECT OF SENESCENCE ON SEROTONERGIC SYSTEMS

Test Subjects	Brain Area	Age of Comparison	Change	Reference
5 - H Y D R O X Y T R Y P T A M I N E			
Human	Hindbrain	25 vs 65 y	0	43
Monkey	Hypothalamus	6 vs 10 y	decrease	42
Mouse	Whole brain	12 vs 28 m	0	41
"	" "	15 vs 28 m	0	48
Chick	Hemisphere	3 vs 3+ m	decrease	49
"	Cerebellum	"	0	49
5 - H Y D R O X Y I N D O L E A C E T I C A C I D			
Human	CSF	30 vs 80 y	+20%	50
"	Hindbrain	25 vs 65 y	0	43
"	"	65 vs 70 y	+30%	43
"	"	25 vs 70 y	0	45
H Y D R O X Y I N D O L E - O - M E T H Y L T R A N S F E R A S E			
Human	Pineal	40-50 vs 55-70 y	-20%	48

TABLE 5

ALTERATIONS IN DOPAMINE ANTAGONIST (SPIROPERIDOL) BINDING SITES IN THE SENESCENT RABBITS[1]

Brain Region	No. of Sites, % Decrease[2] (βmax)	Binding Affinity (K_d)
Caudate-Putamen	35	no change
Frontal Cortex	37	no change
Limbic Cortex	39	no change

[1] Extrapolated from date provided by Makman (personal communication).

[2] Comparison between young and old rabbits.

In the past few years the availability of highly specific CA receptor
ligands have facilitated research on characterizing of those neurotransmitter
receptors. More recently these techniques have been applied in determining
receptor changes related to senescence.

The homogenates of different brain areas obtained from young and old animals have been incubated with a suitable receptor ligand which has previously
been made radioactive so that minute quantities that bind to the receptors can
be traced. Sufficient quantities of the ligand are used to reach binding
equilibrium. The radioactive ligand bound to the receptor membrane is then
differentiated into free and nonspecifically bound quantities. The ligand
specifically bound to the receptor is distinguished from nonspecific binding
by including suitably selected nonradioactive receptor agonists in the incuba-
tion. The stereospecifically active form of these drugs displaces only specifically bound ligand while the biologically nonactive stereoisomer of the
agonist displaces the ligand only from the nonspecific binding sites. This
procedure narrows down most of the bindings to specific receptor sites.

It has been known previously that there is decreased responsiveness to
steroids in aged animals. This was found to be accompanied by a decline in the
number but not in the affinity of steroid receptors in target tissues (for review see 53). Diminished β-adrenergic responsiveness to catecholamines has also
been reported in tissues from senescent rodents and humans (for review see 53).
It has not been well established[53-54] that in senescence there is a decrease
in β-adrenergic receptors in selected brain regions, with greater reduction in
their density seen in the cerebellum, brainstem,pineal gland, and corpus striatum of aged rats, and somewhat lower decrease in the cerebellum of aged humans.
In both rats and humans the decrease is entirely limited to a reduction in the
number of receptor sites with no change reported in receptor affinity. The
cerebral cortex of both rats and humans does not show these changes. It is also known that unlike young animals, the aged rats are unable to increase the
density of adrenergic receptors in response to neuronal hypoactivity.

Data summarized in Table 5 show that there is a significant decrease in the
spiroperidol binding sites in the caudate-putamen, frontal cortex and limbic
cortex of senescent rabbits. Again the decrease is limited entirely to the
binding sites rather than to binding affinity. Similar data have also been obtained from senescent mice and rats where binding sites for both haloperidol
and spiroperidol were shown to be decreased.

The reduction in the binding sites for this CA neurotransmitter is rather
selective as the number of binding sites for benzodiazepines is increased in
aged mice.[55]

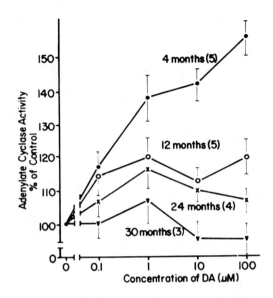

Figure 1. Reduction in dopamine sensitivity of striatal adenylate cyclase related to senescence in the rat. [52]

Alterations in CA neurotransmitter functions is also indicated by pronounced changes in the responsivity of senescent mice to a number of drugs. It has been known for years that the insomniac, anorexent and psychomotor stimulant effects of amphetamine are reduced in the aged. [56-59] Recently it was demonstrated that in aged mice the locomotor stimulant property of dextro-amphetamine was markedly reduced. [36] This is in contrast to another report which showed an increase in the stereotypic response to amphetamine in aged rats. [60] Similarly, sensitivity to the cardiac toxicity of hydralazine is increased in senescence and the lethality due to the direct acting CA drug, phenylephrine, is also enhanced. [61]

CONCLUSION.

Even at this early stage of the neurotransmitter research clear and marked alterations related to senescence have been detected. These changes are profound enough to cause behavioral, cognitive, and endocrinological deficits in the elderly. In addition they are likely to alter responsivity of the elderly to a large number of drugs. However, one must admit that the information presently available is only suggestive and nowhere near adequate to specify clinical applications. A lot more research is needed in the neurotransmitter area to provide rationale approaches to pharmacotherapy in gerentology.

REFERENCES

1. Freund, G. and Walker, D.W. (1971) Life Sci., 10: 1343-1349.
2. Gold, P.E. and McGaugh, J.L. (1975) Neurobiology of Aging, Vol 16
   MS 145-158 in Advances in Behavioral Biology. Eds J.M. Ordy and K.R.
   Brizzee, Plenum Press, New York.
3. Oliverio, A. and Bovet, D. (1966) Life Sci. 5: 1317-1324.
4. Burns, J., Bohdavecky, Z. and Weiss, T. (1962) Psychopharmacologia 3:
   254-262.
5. Stratton, L.O. and Petrinovich, L. (1963) Psychopharmacologia 5: 47-54.
6. Carlton, P.L. and Vogel, J.R. (1965) Psychon. Sci 3: 261-262.
7. Bohdavecky, Z. and Zarvik, M.E. Int. J. Neuropharmacol. 6: 217-222.
8. Dilts, S.L. and Berry, C.A. (1967) J. Pharm. Exp. Ther. 158: 279-285.
9. Moss, D.E. and Deutsch, J.A. (1975) Review of Cholinergic Mechanisms and
   Memory. Ed. P. Wafer 483-492, Raven Press, New York.
10. Drachman, D.A. (1978) Psychopharmacology: A Generation of Progress
    Eds. M.A. Kipton, A.D. Masico, K.F. Killam, Raven Press, New York
    651-652.
11. Hollander, J. and Barrows Jr., C.H. (1968) J. Geront. 23: 174-179.
12. Vakana, T. and Timiras, D.S. (1969) Proc. 8th Int Cong of Gerontology
    Vol. II, 24.
13. Kaur, G. and Kanungo, M.S. (1970) Indian J. Biochem. 7: 122-125.
14. Verkhratsky, A. (1970) Exp. Geront. 5: 4956.
15. McGeer, E.G., Fibiger, H.C., McGeer, P.O. and Wickson, V. (1971) Neurol.
    34: 33-35, Exp. Geront. 6: 391-396.
16. Frolkis, V.V., Bezrukov, V.V., Duplenko, Y.K., Shahegolwa, I.V.,
    Shevtchuk and N.S. Verkhvatsky (1973) Gerontologia 19: 4557.
17. Vasho, M.R., Domino, L.E. and Domino, E.F. (1974) Europ. J. Pharmacol. 72:
    145-147.
18. Meek, J.L., Bertilsson, L., Cheney, D.L., Zsilla, G. and Costa, E. (1977)
    J. Geront. 32: 129-132.
19. Ordy, J.J. and Schjeide, O.A. (1973) Progress in Brain Research Ed. D. H.
    Ford 40: 25-52. Elsevier, New York.
20. Samorajshi, T., Ordy, J.M. and Rady, P. Reinder (1968) Anat. Rec. 16:
    552-562.
21. Vijayar, V.K. (1977) Exp. Geront. 12, 7-11.
22. Haycock, J.W., White, W.F., McGaugh, J.L., Cotman, C.U. (1977). Exp.
    Neurobiol. 57:873-882.
23. Vernadakis, A. (1975) Fed. Proc. 34: 89-95.
24. Samorajshi, T. and C. Rolstein (1973) Progress in Brain Research Ed.
    D.H. Ford 40: 253-266 Elsevier, New York.
25. McGeer, D.L., McGeer, E.C. and Suzuki, J.S. (1977) Arch. Neurol. 34: 33-35.
26. Yamamura, H.J. and Snyder, S.H. (1973) J. Neurochem. 21: 1355-1374.
27. Carroll, P.T. and Butabaugh, G.G. (1975a) J. Neurochem. 24: 229-232.
28. Carroll, P.T. and Butabaugh, G.G. (1975b) J. Neurochem. 24: 917-924.
29. Guyenet, P., Lefresne, P., Rossier, J., Beaujowar, J.C. and Glowinski, J.
    (1973) Molec. Pharmacol. 9: 630-639.
30. Barker, L.A. and Mittag, T.W. (1975) J. Pharm. Exp. Ther. 192: 86-94.
31. Malder, A.H., Yamamura, H.I., Kuhan, M.J. and Snyder, S.H. (1974) Brain
    Res. 70: 372-376.
32. Carroll, P.T. and Goldberg, A.M. (1975) J. Neurochem. 25: 523-527.
33. Richter, J.A. (1976) J. Neurochem. 26: 791-797.
34. Reigine, T.D. Yamamura, H.I., Bird, E.D., Strokes, E. and Enna, S.J.
    (1978) Brain Res. 159: 477-481.
35. Davies, P. and Verth, A.H. (1978) Brain Res. 138: 385-392.
36. Lal, H., Gianforcero, R. and Nandy, K. (1979) Neurosciences Abst. 1979.
37. McGeer, E. and McGeer, P.L. (1976) Neurobiology of Aging, ed. by D.
    Terry, S. Gershon, RavenPress, New York, 389-403.

38. Moore, R. and Bloom, F. Ann. Rev. Neurosci 1: 129-169 (1978)
39. Moore, R. and Bloom, F. Ann. Rev. Neurosci 2: 113-168 (1979).
40. Cote, L.J. and Kremzner, L.T. Transactions of American Society for Neurochemistry, 5th Annual Meeting (1974), New Orleans, LA
41. Finch, C.E. Brain Res. 52: (1973), 261-276.
42. Samorajski, T., Rolsten, C. Prog Brain Res 40: 253-265 (1973).
43. Robinson, D.S., Davis, J.M., Nies, A., Ravaris, C.L., and Sylvester, D. Arch. Gen. Psychiat. 24: 536-539, 1971.
44. Robinson, D.S., Nies, A., Davis, J.N., Bunney, W.E., Davis, J.M., Colburn, R.W., Bourne, H.R., Shaw, D.M. and Coppen, A.J. Lancet 1: 290-291, 1972.
45. Robinson, D.S. Fed. Proc. 34: 103-107, 1975.
46. Bertler, A. Acta Physiol Scand. 51: 97-107, 1961.
47. Wurtman, R.J., Alexrod, J., Barchas, J.D. (1964) J. Clin. Endocrinol. Metab. 24: 299-301.
48. Samorajski, T., Friede, R.L. and Ordy, J.M. (1971) J. Geront. 26: 542-551.
49. Vernadakis, A. (1975) Fed. Proc. 34: 89-95.
50. Gottfries, C.G., Gottfries, I., Johansson, B., Olsson, R., Persoon, T., Ross, B.E., and Sjostrom (1971) Neuropharmacol. 10: 665-672.
51. Zimmerman, I and Berg, A. (1974) Mech. Aging and Dev. 3: 33-36.
52. Puri, S.K. and Volicar, L. (1977) Mech. Aging and Dev. 6: 53-58.
53. Greenberg, L.H. and Weiss, B. (1978). Science 201: 61-63.
54. Maggi, A., Schmidt, M.J., Ghetti, B. and Enna, S.J. (1979) Life Sci. 24: 367-375.
55. Mann, P., Gianforcero, R. and Lal, H.: Life Sci. submitted.
56. Arnett, J.H. and Harris, S.F.: Geriatrics 3: 84-88 (1948).
57. Caveness, W. (1947) N.Y.J. Med., 47: 1003-1005.
58. Krugman, A.D., Ross, S., Vicino, F.L. and Clyde, D.J. (1960) J. Geront. 15: 419-420.
59. Kornetsky, C. (1976). Arch. Gen. Psychiat. 33: 1425-1428.
60. Smith, R.C. and Leelavathi, D.E. (1978) Comm. Psychopharmacol. 2: 39-43.
61. Weiss, L.R. and Krop, S. (1978) In: Pharmacological Intervention in the Aging Process, pp 253-254.

AGE-RELATED FACTORS AFFECTING ANTIDEPRESSANT DRUG METABOLISM
AND CLINICAL RESPONSE

DONALD S. ROBINSON, M.D.
Department of Pharmacology, Marshall University School of Medicine,
Huntington, West Virginia, USA   25701

A variety of genetic, biologic, and environmental factors are known to influence drug metabolism. It has long been appreciated that elderly patients tolerate drugs less well than younger ones[1,2]. There are both pharmacokinetic and pharmacodynamic reasons for this drug intolerance in the older patient. These age-related changes in response to drugs can be due to altered kinetics or to increased receptor sensitivity of target organs[3]. Decreased hepatic microsomal drug metabolizing enzymes with aging has been documented in pharmacokinetic studies[4,5]. This diminished capacity to biotransform drugs accounts in part for some of the difficulties associated with the decreased drug tolerance of the older patient.

Impaired psychotropic drug metabolism with advancing age has been reported for several drugs, including the widely-used benzodiazepine anti-anxiety agents[6-8] and the antidepressants[9,10]. This diminished ability to metabolize many psychotropic drugs with advancing age has only recently been appreciated. There is now convincing evidence that the pharmacokinetics of nearly all the benzodiazepine and barbiturate sedative-hypnotics are affected by age[6,11,12]. Their diminished rate of biotransformation is presumably due to a gradual decline in the specific activities of microsomal drug metaboliz-ing enzymes, as well as possibly due to a loss of liver mass in relation to body size with aging. Impairment of liver function with congestive heart failure and diminished renal function with advancing age can also contribute to decreased drug and metabolite clearance. Whatever the mechanism of this impaired metabolism, the older patient is predictably more likely to develop toxic plasma and tissue drug levels at what would be standard doses of psychopharmacologic drugs in younger patients.

Excessive tricyclic antidepressant (TCA) blood and tissue levels may partially account for the increased susceptibility of elderly patients to

TCA side effects. This is a particular concern with TCA therapy because of their significant and occasionally toxic cardiac effects[13,14].

Altered clinical efficacy of antidepressant drugs in the older age groups is another largely unstudied question. Adequate clinical trials of antidepressant and other psychoactive drugs in the elderly as a separate and distinct population, are lacking as a basis for rational psychopharmacologic therapy. Emphasis on aging research has only recently focused investigative attention on the special therapeutic problems of the elderly. It will predictably be several years before the results of studies in progress in this area will be available for clinical application.

The inherent difficulties of antidepressant drug trials is further compounded in aged populations by the added complexities of diagnosis, problems with the recognition of pseudodementia, and the confounding of symptomatology by concomitant medical and neurological illnesses and drugs with CNS side effects. Because of uncertainties about the diagnosis of depressive illness in the elderly and the poorer tolerance of the older patient to antidepressant drugs, clinicians are often reluctant to initiate antidepressant drug treatment even when it is likely to be beneficial. When the clinician does prescribe an antidepressant in this setting, there are few guidelines as to proper dose, appropriate clinical endpoints, and therapeutic expectations.

In this chapter, I shall review recent research findings relative to aging effects on antidepressant metabolism and clinical response to both the tricyclic and MAO inhibitor antidepressant drugs in the elderly.*

TRICYCLIC ANTIDEPRESSANT DRUGS

In a preliminary study, we reported from our laboratory that plasma TCA half-lives and steady state levels are positively correlated with age in patients treated with imipramine or amitriptyline[9]. We have now extended these findings of an age relationship to a larger patient sample. Plasma TCA levels were measured at steady state in 40 patients treated in an outpatient trial for six weeks with amitriptyline 150 mg/day. Blood levels were obtained every two weeks during the six week treatment period, and in all cases, steady state was achieved by four weeks. The four-week values were

---

*Studies cited in this chapter were carried out in collaboration with A. Nies, Marshall University School of Medicine, Huntington, West Virginia, T.B. Cooper, Rockland Research Institute, Orangeburg, New York, and C.L. Ravaris, Eastern Carolina University, Greenville, North Carolina.

used in the analysis. We also studied an inpatient population treated on a hospital psychiatric service with imipramine for varying periods of time. Most of these patients received imipramine 150 mg/day for at least three weeks, and the plasma disappearance half-life study was measured when the drug was discontinued after steady state conditions had been achieved. Patients with serious underlying medical illness, including acute alcoholism, liver dysfunction, etc., were excluded from the analysis. The 40 outpatients in the amitriptyline study ranged from 21 to 68 years of age, and the 25 imipramine-treated patients from 27 to 78 years. None of the patients were receiving other concurrent psychotropic medications. The only permitted drugs other than the antidepressant were chloral hydrate if necessary for sleep and aspirin or acetaminophen for headache or pain. Plasma concentrations of amitriptyline, imipramine, and their demethylated metabolites were determined by a gas chromatographic method with a coefficient variation of $\pm5\%$ across the concentration range of 5-250 ng/ml[15]. Imipramine elimination half-lives and desipramine disappearance half-lives ($T\frac{1}{2}$) were calculated using a standard program for fitting a logarithmic decay curve in linear form. It can be seen in the following table (Table 1) that both imipramine and amitriptyline steady state plasma levels correlated significantly with age.

TABLE 1

CORRELATION OF STEADY STATE PLASMA CONCENTRATIONS (C_{ss}) AND DISAPPEARANCE HALF-LIVES ($T\frac{1}{2}$) WITH AGE IN IMIPRAMINE AND AMITRIPTYLINE-TREATED PATIENTS

	Correlation Coefficient (r)	
	C_{ss} vs. Age	$T\frac{1}{2}$ vs. Age
Imipramine	+ .46* (n=22)	+ .21 (n=25)
Desipramine	+ .18	+ .51**
Amitriptyline	+ .45*** (n=40)	———
Nortriptyline	+ .01	———

*p < .05
**p < .01
***p < .005

On the other hand, their respective demethylated metabolites, nortriptyline and desipramine, did not show a significant correlation of steady state plasma levels with age. A possible interpretation of this finding is that

N-demethylation, a major metabolic pathway for the tertiary compounds, becomes less efficient with aging. This would be consistent with reports that microsomal drug metabolism enzymes show an age-related decline in activity in man[4,5].

The disappearance $T\frac{1}{2}$ of desipramine in patients treated with imipramine, however, did show a significant positive correlation with age. This could be accounted for by decreased clearance of desipramine, by altered pharmacokinetics of the parent compound, imipramine, or both. The steady state elimination $T\frac{1}{2}$ of imipramine was not significantly prolonged although there was a trend toward a positive correlation with age (r = + .21).

The plasma $T\frac{1}{2}$ values for patients above and below 50 years of age in a group of non-smokers and non-drinkers were examined. The older patients did have significantly longer imipramine and desipramine $T\frac{1}{2}$'s (Table 2) with the mean disappearance $T\frac{1}{2}$ for desipramine in the over 50 years group being markedly prolonged with a large variance.

TABLE 2

PLASMA DISAPPEARANCE HALF-LIVES ($T\frac{1}{2}$) OF IMIPRAMINE AND DESIPRAMINE OF PATIENTS ABOVE AND BELOW 50 YEARS OF AGE

	Mean Plasma $T\frac{1}{2}$ (hrs.)†	
	< 50 Years (n=8)	≥ 50 Years (n=8)
Imipramine	18.5 ± 3.4	23.2 ± 1.4*
Desipramine	35.9 ± 2.9	55.8 ± 11.9*

†Mean $T\frac{1}{2}$ ± SEM for non-smokers treated with imipramine 150 mg/day for 3 weeks
*Difference between mean $T\frac{1}{2}$ for young and old patients significant at P < .05

Since dosage (mg/kg of body weight) can also be a determinant of plasma TCA levels, relationships between age and body weight were examined for both the amitriptyline-treated and the imipramine-treated patients. Body weight did not correlate with age in either patient group. Thus, the possibility that the age related differences in steady state levels are attributable to a higher dosage (mg/kg) in the older patients has been excluded.

The age-related changes in TCA pharmacokinetics cited here extend our previous findings in a smaller series of patients[9] and suggest that the aging process is an important determinant of biotransformation in addition

to genetically determined interindividual differences in TCA levels and
$T\frac{1}{2}$'s. As much as 20% of the variance of steady state plasma levels of
imipramine and amitriptyline may be accountable by this apparent aging
effect on TCA metabolism.

Other environmental factors are also known to be important in the
metabolism of TCAs and other drugs. Chronic alcohol users tend to have
shorter TCA half-lives than non-drinkers. Similarly, we and others[16] find
that smokers metabolize imipramine more rapidly than non-smokers. It is
likely that other environmental and dietary factors also have important
influences on drug metabolism. These include interacting drugs, which can
either stimulate or inhibit metabolism, ingestion of trace hydrocarbons in
diet, as well as cigarette smoking all of which may induce liver microsomal
enzymes.

Aging and Clinical Response to Amitriptyline

In a recent double blind clinical comparison of amitriptyline and
phenelzine in depressed outpatients, we examined treatment response and drug
side effects as a function of age. Sixty-six patients ranging in age from
20 to 67 years with significant depressive symptoms were treated with amitriptyline after a one week drug free control period. Patients treated
with amitriptyline received 75 mg/day for the first five days, then 150
mg/day for the remainder of the six week drug treatment period. Most patients were maintained on this fixed dosage although a decrease in dose to
125 or 100 mg/day was permitted if suspected side effects were severe.

Fifteen of the 66 amitriptyline-treated patients admitted to the protocol dropped out, mostly because of failure to respond. The overall amitriptyline response rate proved to be 54% (patients showing marked improvement
in the total sample including dropouts). Drug response as judged by global
improvement rated by the psychiatrist who remained blind to drug assignment
was relatively constant across the age spectrum. There was not a significant
association of global improvement rate with age for these 66 patients (Kendall's tau = -.02).

The only clinical predictor of amitriptyline response in this outpatient population was the 17-item Hamilton Depression Score (HDS) at baseline. The more severely symptomatic patients on endogenous items (high HDS)
tended to show better response to tricyclic antidepressant than those with
less severity on endogenous items.

We also examined for relationships of amitriptyline dosage (mg/kg) or plasma TCA levels with clinical drug effects. Amitriptyline dosage (mg/kg) showed no relationship to either global improvement or change scores on structured depression interview items. Similarly, there was no relationship of plasma amitriptyline, nortriptyline, or total TCA levels to clinical response or side effects[17].

We also examined the incidence of side effects in TCA-treated patients as a function of age. It can be seen in the Table 3 that older outpatients tended to have fewer side effects during treatment with amitriptyline 150 mg/day than younger patients despite the fact that plasma TCA concentrations tend to be higher with increasing age.

TABLE 3

SIDE EFFECTS DURING AMITRIPTYLINE TREATMENT: RELATIONSHIP TO AGE

Age	Dry Mouth	Sedation	Faintness	Total No. Side Effects per Patient
< 50 yrs.	38/42*	18/42	25/42	3.4 ± 0.3*
> 50 yrs.	7/13	4/12	7/13	2.8 ± 0.6

* Patients < 50 yrs. reported higher incidence of side effects, p < .05.

Adverse central nervous system effects of TCAs manifested by confusional episodes in the elderly have been clinically recognized but difficult to document. Davies and Associates[18] noted that 13% of patients overall receiving TCAs exhibited confusion but that confusional episodes occurred in 35% of the patients over 40 years of age. The tendency for older patients to develop higher steady state TCA levels may in part account for these observations. Although in our clinical trial there were only 13 patients between the ages of 50 and 69 years treated with amitriptyline, it is interesting that we did not observe any confusional episodes or other more troublesome side effects (Table 3). None of our patients exhibited manifestations of pseudodementia, but this problem may be less likely in an outpatient sample such as ours.

Clinicians often have difficulty in distinguishing contribution of drug and underlying illness to the appearance of organic signs in their elderly patients. In many cases, downward adjustment of TCA dosage might be the correct therapeutic decision in such situations where toxic levels are somewhat more probable rather than doubting the diagnosis of depressive illness and incorrectly discontinuing antidepressant drug treatment when it is still indicated.

Because of longer elimination T½'s, there will be a significant number of elderly patients who do not achieve steady state TCA levels within the first five to seven days of treatment as is usually the case for younger patients. Thus in many older patients, steady state may not be achieved for ten to fourteen days, or longer in the occasional patient, and the full effects of antidepressant drug treatment may be very delayed. The typical 10-21 day lag before significant antidepressant response to TCA is evident may be even longer in the patient 60 years of age or older, especially when appropriately reduced starting doses are used.

It is probably prudent to reduce standard TCA dosage in the patient over 60 years of age by 30 to 50% from that usually recommended. In the case of imipramine, it is suggested that treatment be initiated with 25 mg/day at bed time, with progressive increments every 4-7 days until 100 mg/day is reached or troublesome side effects intervene, whichever occurs first.

MONAMINE OXIDASE INHIBITORS

Recently, there has been a resurgence of interest in the MAO inhibiting (MAOI) antidepressant drugs. This has been due to several factors, including the often troublesome side effects of TCAs in both young and old patients, and concern about the lower tolerance to the cardiovascular and anticholinergic effects of TCAs in the elderly. Lack of uniformly favorable therapeutic response to TCAs has also generated interest in defining MAOI responsive patients, and in using MAOIs in patients who do not respond to TCA treatment. It is possible that many elderly depressed patients may show suboptimal response to TCAs because of greater intolerance in general to side effects, or depressive illness in the elderly may be generally more refractory to drug treatment. These issues will require elucidation, and adequate studies in the appropriate age groups in geriatric populations are lacking to clarify these points.

The MAOIs continued to be used in other countries, particularly the United Kingdom when popularity declined in this country in the early 1960's. Early reports of their effectiveness in so-called atypical depressions aroused little interest in the U.S. until recent years. Comprehensive clinical investigations of the MAOIs were not performed until recently because of their general unpopularity. Thus, until recently, MAOIs were regarded as basically second or third line drugs for use in resistant depressions.

A number of controlled clinical trials[20-24] have now documented significant antidepressant and antiphobic activity for the MAOI, phenelzine. These tend to suggest that the clinical indication for MAOI treatment are for nonendogenous depressions and phobic-anxiety states[25].

Relatively little is known about the efficacy of MAOI drugs in the older age groups. We have recently examined the data from three double blind controlled clinical trials of phenelzine with respect to age and therapeutic effect[20,22,26].

We originally reported in 1971 a significant age-MAO relationship in blood platelets, plasma, and brain from human subjects[27]. There was a significant positive correlation of age and MAO activity in all three tissues. Furthermore, women had significantly higher mean MAO activity than men, suggesting that sex, in addition to age, might be a biologic determinant of enzyme activity. Additional human brain studies reported in 1977 again confirmed the MAO-age relationship in eight areas of human brain[28]. In data from our clinical trials of phenelzine, we see a significant blood platelet MAO-age relationship in depressed outpatients, replicating the findings of the previously cited studies and strongly suggesting that increased catabolism of biogenic amines may be a phenomenon of aging. Table 4 shows mean blood platelet MAO activities as a function of age and sex from these clinical trials[20,22,26].

TABLE 4

PLATELET MAO ACTIVITY† BY AGE DECADE AND SEX IN DEPRESSED OUTPATIENTS FROM THREE CONTROLLED CLINICAL TRIALS PRIOR TO ANTIDEPRESSANT DRUG TREATMENT

Age (yr)	20-29	30-39	40-49	50-59	60-69	Total
Men	14.7±9.8	20.0±11.9	24.9±9.2	24.3±14.6	31.8±15.8	21.6±12.6
(n)	15	22	14	17	5	73
Women	31.8±17.7	31.7±16.6	29.2±16.3	30.0±14.9	43.1±19.0	32.3±17.0
(n)	39	68	40	28	20	198

†Mean ± SEM of platelet MAO activity with benzylamine substrate, expressed as nmol/mg protein/hr.

Aging and Clinical Response to Phenelzine

Since elderly patients on the average have higher MAO activity in a number of tissues including brain, this finding suggests the possibility that MAOIs might be preferentially more efficacious in treating depressive illnesses in older patients. Consequently, we have examined the clinical response rate to the two antidepressants, phenelzine and amitriptyline, in our three previously reported trials[20,22,26]. It can be seen in Table 5 that global improvement scores (by blind psychiatrist evaluation) showed a progressively better response rate in the phenelzine-treated group with increasing age. The response rates shown include completers and dropouts so that overall response rates to antidepressant drug treatment appear somewhat lower than customarily stated. It can also be seen by comparison that the amitriptyline response rate was not significantly influenced by age.

TABLE 5

AGE VS. ANTIDEPRESSANT DRUG RESPONSE RATE†

Age	Amitriptyline Response Rate (%)	n	Phenelzine Response* Rate (%)	n
< 30 yrs.	50%	18	26%	31
30 < 45	57	28	54	67
45 < 60	25	16	56	36
> 60	60	5	69	13

† % patients (including dropouts) markedly improved by blind global rating after 6 weeks treatment with amitriptyline 150 mg/day or phenelzine 60 mg/day.
* Phenelzine responders are significantly older than non-responders ($p < .01$).

Since response to phenelzine has previously been shown to require an approximately 80% inhibition of platelet MAO[20,22,26], one could ask whether the better response in older patients was due to greater inhibition of the platelet enzyme. We examined the correlations of age and percent of platelet MAO inhibition with both benzylamine and tryptamine as substrates and found them to be non-significant ($r = -.11$ and $-.02$, respectively). Not surprisingly, patient weight did correlate significantly with percent inhibition ($r = -.54$ for benzylamine, $p < .005$; and $r = -.47$ for tryptamine, $p < .01$). There was no correlation between patient age and weight.

The recent development of a sensitive assay for phenelzine[30] has allowed us to examine plasma drug levels as well as platelet MAO inhibition during phenelzine therapy. In 55 phenelzine-treated patients from our current phenelzine-amitriptyline clinical trial[27,29], we found a weak positive correlation of plasma phenelzine level with age. This age-drug level correlation tends to disappear after two weeks of drug treatment while a strong positive correlation subsequently develops between dosage (mg/kg) and plasma phenelzine level. Percent platelet MAO inhibition and plasma phenelzine concentration are also significantly correlated as shown in Table 6.

TABLE 6

CORRELATION (r) OF PHENELZINE PLASMA LEVELS WITH AGE, PERCENT MAO INHIBITION, AND GLOBAL IMPROVEMENT

Duration of Treatment (wk)	Age (r)	%MAO Inhibition† (r)	Global Improvement (Kendall's tau)
2	+ .32*	+ .21*	- .06
4	+ .16	+ .46**	+ .15
6	+ .14	+ .30**	+ .26*

†Inhibition of platelet MAO activity, with tryptamine as substrate.
*p < .05.
**p < .01.

Plasma phenelzine levels also correlate at 6 weeks of phenelzine treatment with improvement on several major symptom scales of the structured depression interview, including the 17-item Hamilton Depression Scale (r = +.33, p < .01). The tendency for somewhat higher plasma phenelzine levels in the older patients and the greater clinical response to MAOI in these patients might be accounted for by a slowing of phenelzine metabolism and clearance. We examined rate of drug acetylation in the phenelzine-treated patients. Acetylation phenotyping was carried out in 40 patients from our phenelzine controlled clinical trials using sulfapyridine according to the method of Price Evans[31]. This acetylator phenotyping identified 25 slow and 15 fast acetylators. Interestingly, we found no relationship between rate of drug acetylation and clinical improvement or percent platelet MAO inhibition. Also, rate of drug acetylation did not appear to be influenced by aging. These findings do not support the suggestion that acetylation is a major determinant of phenelzine metabolism. Also it might be regarded as evidence that the non-microsomal enzyme, acetyl transferase, like MAO does not diminish in activity with aging. This is consistent with recent study by Farah et al.[32] who found isoniazid half-lives to be unaffected by age, while acetanilide half-lives were significantly prolonged in the elderly.

SUMMARY

This paper has reviewed some of the recent pharmacokinetic, biologic, and clinical data relating to aging and antidepressant drugs. Considerably more work must be done to delineate the appropriate therapeutic role of each antidepressant drug class in elderly populations and in different diagnostic categories. There is evidence that biotransformation of the tricyclic antidepressant drugs is slowed in the elderly and significantly modified doses should be employed in these populations. The MAO inhibiting drugs have been relatively unstudied in the aged. The preliminary evidence suggests they may have particular efficacy in the older patients perhaps due to enhanced MAO activity with advancing age and the intolerance of many elderly patients to tricyclic antidepressants.

ACKNOWLEDGEMENTS

This research was supported in part by the Burroughs Wellcome Fund and US Public Health Service grant, MH 15533, and was carried out in collaboration with Alexander Nies, M.D., Department of Psychiatry, Marshall University School of Medicine, Huntington, WV, T. B. Cooper, M.S., Rockland Research Institute, Orangeburg, NY 10962, and C. Lewis Ravaris, Ph.D., M.D., Department of Psychiatry, East Carolina School of Medicine, Greenville, NC 27834.

REFERENCES

1. Smith, J.W., Seidl, L.G., and Cluff, L.E. (1966) Studies on the epidemiology of adverse drug reactions: V. Clinical factors influencing susceptibility. Ann. Intern. Med. 65, 629-640.
2. Hurwitz, N. (1969) Predisposing factors in adverse reactions to drugs. Br. Med. J. 1, 536-539.
3. Bender, A.D. (1974) Pharmacodynamic principles of drug therapy in the aged. J. Am. Geriat. Soc. 23, 296-303.
4. O'Malley, K., Crooks, J., Duke, E., and Stevenson, I.H. (1971) Effect of age and sex in human drug metabolism. Br. Med. J. 3, 607-609.
5. Vestal, R.E., Norris, A.H., Tobin, J.D., Cohen, B.H., Shock, N.W., and Andres, R. (1975) Antipyrine metabolism in man: Influence of age, alcohol, caffeine, and smoking. Clin. Pharmacol. Ther. 18, 425-432.
6. Greenblatt, D.J., Harmatz, J.S., and Shader, R.I. (1978) Factors influencing diazepam pharmacokinetics: Age, sex, and liver disease. Int. J. Clin. Pharmacol. and Biopharm. 16 (4):177-179.
7. Greenblatt, D.J., Allen, M.D., and Shader, R.I. (1977) Toxicity of high dose flurazepam in the elderly. Clin. Pharmacol. Ther. 21, 355-361.

8. Greenblatt, D.J., Harmatz, J.S., Stanski, D.R., and Shader, R.I. (1977) Factors influencing blood concentrations of chlordiazepoxide: A case for multiple regression analyses. Psychopharmacology 54, 277-282.

9. Nies, A., Robinson, D.S., Friedman, M.J., Green, R., Cooper, T.B., Ravaris, C.L., and Ives, J.O. (1977) Relationship between age and tricyclic antidepressant plasma levels. Am. J. Psychiat. 134, 790-793.

10. Gram, L.F., Sondergaard, I.B., Christiansen, J., Peterson, G.O., Bech, P., Reisby, N., Ibsen, I., Ortmann, J., Nagy, A., Dencker, S.J., Jacobsen, O., and Krautwald, O. (1977) Steady-state kinetics of imipramine in patients. Psychopharmacology 54, 255-261.

11. Klotz, U., Avanti, G.R., Hoyumpa, A., Schenker, S., and Wilkinson, G.R. (1975) The effects of age and liver disease on the disposition and elimination of diazepam in man. J. Clin. Invest. 55, 347-359.

12. Irvine, R.E., Grove, J., Toseland, P.A., Trounce, P.A., Jr. (1974) Effect of age on the hydroxylation of amylobarbitone sodium in man. Br. J. Clin. Pharmacol. 1, 41-43.

13. Robinson, D.S. and Barker, E. (1976) Tricyclic antidepressant cardiotoxicity. J.A.M.A. 236, 2089-2090.

14. Kantor, S.J., Glassman, A.H., Bigger, J.T., Perel, J.M., and Giardina, E.V. (1978) The cardiac effects of therapeutic concentrations of imipramine. Am. J. Psychiat. 135, 534-538.

15. Cooper, T.B., Allen, D., and Simpson, G.M. (1976) A sensitive method for the determination of amitriptyline and nortriptyline in human plasma. Psychopharmacol. Comm. 2, 105-116.

16. Perel, J.M., Shostak, M., Gann, E., Kantor, S.J., and Glassman, A.H. (1976) Pharmacodynamics of imipramine and clinical outcome in depressed patients. In: Pharmacokinetics of Psychoactive Drugs: Blood Levels and Clinical Response, L.S. Gottschalk and S. Merlin, eds., Spectrum Publications, New York, pp. 229-241.

17. Robinson, D.S., Cooper, T.B., Ravaris, C.L., Ives, J.O., Nies, A., Bartlett, D.B., and Lamborn, K.R. (1979) Plasma tricyclic drug levels in amitriptyline-treated depressed patients. Psychopharmacology, in press.

18. Davies, R.K., Tucker, G.J., Harrow, M., and Detre, T.P. (1971) Confusional episodes and autidepressant medication. Am. J. Psychiat. 181, 127-131.

19. West, E.D. and Dally, P.J. (1959) Effects of isoniazid in depressive syndromes. Br. Med. J. 1, 1491-1494.

20. Robinson, D.S., Nies, A., Ravaris, C.L., and Lamborn, K.R. (1973) The monoamine oxidase inhibitor, phenelzine, in the treatment of depressive-anxiety states. Arch. Gen. Psychiat. 29, 407-413.

21. Johnstone, E.C. and Marsh, W. (1973) Acetylator status and response to phenelzine in depressed patients. Lancet 1, 567-570.

22. Ravaris, C.L., Nies, A., Robinson, D.S., Ives, J.O., Lamborn, K.R., and Korson, L. (1976) A multiple-dose, controlled study of phenelzine in depression-anxiety states. Arch. Gen. Psychiat. 33, 347-350.

23. Tyrer, P., Candy, J., and Kelly, D. (1973) Phenelzine in phobic anxiety: A controlled trial. Psychol. Med. 3, 120-124.

24. Ballenger, J., Sheehan, D., and Jacobson, G. (1977) Drug treatment of agoraphobia. Paper presented at the annual meeting, American Psychiatric Association, Toronto, May, 1977.

25. Nies, A., Robinson, D.S., Lamborn, K.R., Ravaris, C.L., and Ives, J.O. (1975) The efficacy of the MAO inhibitor, phenelzine: Dose effects and prediction of response. In: Neuropsychopharmacology, Excerpta Medica Press, Amsterdam, pp. 765-770.

26. Robinson, D.S., Nies, A., Ravaris, C.L., Ives, J.O., and Bartlett, D. (1978) Clinical pharmacology of phenelzine. Arch. Gen. Psychiat. 35, 629-635.

27. Robinson, D.S., Davis, J.M., Nies, A., Ravaris, C.L., and Sylwester, D. (1971) Relation of sex and aging to monoamine oxidase activity of human brain, plasma, and platelets. Arch. Gen. Psychiat. 24, 536-539.

28. Robinson, D.S., Sourkes, T.L., Nies, A., Harris, L.S., Spector, S., Bartlett, D.L., and Kaye, I.S. (1977) Monoamine metabolism in human brain. Arch. Gen. Psychiat. 34, 89-92.

29. Ravaris, C.L., Robinson, D.S., Ives, J.O., Nies, A., and Bartlett, D. (1979) A comparison of phenelzine and amitriptyline in the treatment of depression. Arch. Gen. Psychiat., in press.

30. Cooper, T.B., Robinson, D.S., and Nies, A. (1978) Phenelzine measurement in human plasma: A sensitive GLC-ECD procedure. Comm. in Psychopharmacol. 2, 502-512.

31. Price Evans, D.A. (1969) An improved and simplified method of detecting the acetylator phenotype. J. Med. Genet. 6, 405-407.

32. Farah, F., Taylor, W., Rawlins, M.D., and James. O. (1977) Hepatic drug acetylation and oxidation: Effects of aging in man. Br. Med. J. 2, 155-156.

Published 1979 by Elsevier North Holland, Inc.
Nandy, Ed. Geriatric Psychopharmacology

AGE-RELATED CHANGE IN THE PHARMACOKINETICS OF SOME PSYCHOTROPHIC DRUGS

AND ITS CLINICAL IMPLICATIONS

Zafar H. Israili, Ph.D.
Departments of Medicine and Chemistry
Emory University School of Medicine
Atlanta, GA 30322

INTRODUCTION

Psychoactive drugs are among the therapuetic agents more frequently prescrib-ed for the elderly[1-3] and these drugs are reported to cause adverse effects in an excessive portion of patients.[4] In a review of the hospital usage of drugs, out of a total of 1,431 chronically ill elderly patients, psychoactive drugs had been prescribed for about one quarter of the patients[5] and mostly to provide night-time sedation.

The benzodiazepines (Table 1) are among the most widely used drugs in the world in the treatment of insomnia, anxiety, seizures and alcoholism. Although benzodiazepines possess a wide margin of therapeutic safety, their use is not without a considerable incidence of side effects.[6-11] The extensive prescribing of these drugs for elderly patients has generated considerable concern.[2,4,12,13]

An increased frequency of adverse reactions including cardiovascular compli-cations, hypotension, unacceptable central nervous system depression attributed to several benzodiazepine hypnotics in elderly patients has been reported.[8,14-16] A similar association of toxicity with increasing age has not been found for nonbenzodiazepine hypnotics, such as chloral hydrate and barbiturates.[17]

TABLE 1

BENZODIAZEPINES

DRUG	R_1	R_2	R_3	X	Y	Z
DIAZEPAM (Valium and others)	Cl	H	–	CH_3	=0	H
DESMETHYLDIAZEPAM	Cl	H	–	H	=0	H
TEMAZEPAM	Cl	H	–	CH_3	=0	OH
OXAZEPAM (Serax)	Cl	H	–	H	=0	OH
CHLORDIAZEPOXIDE* (Librium and others)	Cl	H	0	–	$-N \begin{smallmatrix} H \\ CH_3 \end{smallmatrix}$	H
DESMETHYL CHLOR-* DIAZEPOXIDE	Cl	H	0	–	$-NH_2$	H
DEMOXEPAM	Cl	H	0	H	=0	H
FLURAZEPAM (Dalmane)	Cl	F	–	$-(CH_2)_2N(C_2H_5)_2$	=0	H
NITRAZEPAM (Mogadon)	NO_2	H	–	H	=0	H
CHLORAZEPATE DIPOTASSIUM (Tranxene)	Cl	H	–	H	$\langle \begin{smallmatrix} OH \\ O^-K^+ \end{smallmatrix}$	$-COO^-K^+$
LORAZEPAM (Ativan)	Cl	Cl	–	H	=0	OH

*double bond between positions 1 and 2

TABLE 2

AGE-RELATED CHANGES AFFECTING THE PHARMACOKINETICS OF DRUGS

Organ	Physiological Change	Major Effect	Pharmacokinetic Consequence
Gastrointestinal tract	Atrophic changes in mucosa, decreased intestinal and splan-chnic blood flow; de-creased acid secre-tion in stomach	Decreased transport efficiency	Decreased and/or delayed absorption of drugs
Kidney	Thickening of base-ment membrane of Bowman's capsule; impaired permeabi-lity; decreased renal blood flow	Decreased Glomerular filtration rate and maximum excretory capacity	Decreased clearance and increased plasma elimination half-life of drugs
Liver	Decreased hepatic blood flow Decreased metabo-lizing enzymes	Decreased availability of drugs to the liver	Decreased metabolism and increased plasma elimination half-life of drugs
Plasma	Decreased proteins	Decreased binding	Higher levels of free drug in plasma
Muscle	Decreased muscle mass; more fat	Altered dis-tribution	Altered apparent volume and distri-bution and plasma elimination of some drugs

The efficacy of lithium in the treatment of psychotic and manic-depressive illness is well established.[18-20] The potential for toxicity of lithium in the elderly is fairly high.

Recognition of potential unwanted effects of these drugs and of factors pre-disposing to toxicity are important to insure appropriate use in clinical medi-cine.

Aging is generally associated with many physiological and biochemical changes which affect tissue reactivity, sensitivity, and tolerance to drugs by modifi-cation of the drug action at the molecular level. The altered response to

various drugs in the elderly could be due to age-related modification of the
site(s) of action and/or modification of the pharmacokinetic profile of a drug
(caused by functional change, Table 2) resulting in altered levels of free drug
at its site(s) of action.

The age-related pharmacokinetics of a number of benzodiazepines and lithium
and the probable mechanism(s) of increased response of these drugs in the elderly are reviewed.

ALTERATION IN THE ABSORPTION, DISTRIBUTION, METABOLISM AND EXCRETION OF DRUGS
IN AGING

Absorption

Aging may modify the absorption of drugs from the gastrointestinal tract in
a number of ways: 1) Decreased secretion of acid in the stomach results in
elevated gastric pH which in turn increases gastric motility; the absorption of acidic drugs is expected to decrease while that of basic drugs is to
be favored. 2) Reduction in intestinal blood flow. Although it has been reported that intestinal and splanchnic blood flow is decreased,[21,22] there are
no systematic studies to support it; this decrease has been assumed on the
basis of age-related reduction (30-40% attenuation between the ages of 25 and
65 years) in cardiac output.[21,23] 3) Reduction in the number of absorbing cells
and surface area. There is insufficient data to permit an estimate of changes
in the number of absorbing cells in the intestine. In a recent study,[24] evidence was presented that the mucosal surface area was significantly reduced in
the well-nourished elderly subjects (60-73 years) as compared to that in the
younger group (16-30 years).

So far, there is little evidence, supported by systematic studies, to suggest that any major alteration occurs in the absorption of drugs (most of which
are absorbed passively) from the gastrointestinal tract as a result of aging.[25]
Increased plasma levels of some drugs in the elderly, as compared to that in
the young subjects (e.g. acetaminophen, sulfamethizole, propranolol) has been

rationalized on the basis of decreased elimination rate and/or reduction in the apparent volume of distribution.[25,26] The rate of absorption of chlordia- zepoxide[27], digoxin[28] and lorazepam[29] has been reported to be much slower in the elderly than in the younger subjects. The absorption of chlorazepate di- potassium may be decreased in the elderly because of the lower amount of acid normally secreted in the stomach with aging, and since absorption of this drug depends on the presence of acid in the stomach[30].

Distribution

Elderly patients, in general, have smaller muscle mass and total body wa- ter.[31] Much of the metabolically active tissue is replaced by fat. Body fat increases from 18 to 36% of total body weight in men and from 33 to 48% in women as the age increases from 18 to 55 years.[32] Consequently, highly lipid soluble drugs may accumulate and have longer duration of action. Nevertheless, there is no consistent pattern of age-related changes in terms of distribution pattern or volume.

The apparent volume of distribution in the elderly has been found to be larger than that in young subjects for some drugs: diazepam[33], chlordiaze- poxide[27,34], nitrazepam[35] and lower for some: antipyrine[36] and propicillin[37]. However, in the case of acetaminophen and phenylbutazone[38], warfarin[39], sulfa- methizole[38] and flurazepam[40], there was no age-related change in the volume of distribution. For some benzodiazepines, the weight corrected volume of distribution for women is greater than in men[41] (since women have a higher fat/muscle ratio and also because of different pattern of protein), suggesting greater uptake by tissues in women.

Plasma protein binding. The levels of plasma proteins also change with age; generally the albumin level falls and gamma globulin concentration increases.[42] In a recent survey by Greenblatt[43] involving more than 11,000 patients, it was reported that mean serum albumin concentration fell progressively with each decade of age. At age $\leq$ 40 years, the concentration was 3.97 g/100 ml while at age $\geqslant$ 80 years, the concentration was 3.58 g/100 ml; this difference was found to be significant. The reduced serum albumin concentration in the elderly could contribute to age-dependent changes in the binding and apparent volume of distribution of some drugs; these changes in turn can influence the clinical effects of the drugs.

Significant age-related decrease in plasma protein binding of several drugs has been reported: phenytoin[44,45], warfarin[45], meperidine[46] and phenylbutazone[47]; for some drugs there was no change e.g. diazepam[33], desmethyldiazepam[33], salicylate[47], sulfadiazine[47], chlordiazepoxide[34], phenobarbital[48] and penicillin[48].

Most studies of pharmacokinetic changes associated with aging have focussed on total rather than unbound concentration of drug in plasma or serum; the pharmacokinetic parameters should be calculated on the basis of free drug in plasma.

Binding to red cells. There may be some age-related alteration in the binding of drugs to red cells. For example, Chan et al.[49] demonstrated that higher levels of meperidine in the plasma of the elderly was due to decreased binding of the drug to red cells (25%) when compared with that of young patients (50%). No such age-related differences in red cell binding were found for pentazocine[50] and diazepam[33].

Metabolism

Age-related changes in metabolism may be due to alteration in liver blood flow and/or a change in hepatic drug metabolizing enzymes.

Aging and liver blood flow. The hepatic blood flow is diminished in the elderly. Bender[21] reviewed published reports on the effects of increasing age on peripheral blood flow and concluded that regional blood flow was not uniformly affected. Whereas cardiac output decreases, the cerebral, coronary and skeletal blood flow tended to be maintained at the expense of supply to other organs including the liver. As the cardiac output decreases by about

30%, the hepatic flow is reduced by about 40-50% at the age of 60,when compared to that in individuals averaging 25 years.[22] This decrease was also suggested from several studies carried out with propranolol.[51-53]

Aging and liver drug metabolizing enzymes. The early studies of Kato and co-workers demostrated that aging rats have lower than normal hepatic microsomal drug metabolizing activity, lower liver cytochrome P-450 content and that they respond relatively poorly to enzyme-inducing agents.[54-56]

There are no published data describing age-related changes in the microsomal drug metabolizing enzyme activity in man. Results from a number of studies using indirect methods indicate that elderly subjects may have a reduced ability to metabolize a number of drugs including antipyrine, aminopyrine, amylobarbital, acetaminophen, phenylbutazone, warfarin, phenytoin, diazepam and indomethacin.[25,57,58] These drugs are metabolized via the liver microsomal mixed function oxidase system. The evidence for decreased metabolism has been obtained from determination of the plasma elimination half-life (significantly higher)and/or plasma clearance (lower in the elderly than in the younger population). In some cases, the excretion(and maybe the formation) of metabolites has been shown to be decreased in the elderly.

Excretion

Many drugs are eliminated by the kidneys and for some (e.g. many antibiotics and some cardiac glycosides) it may be the exclusive route of elimination. Therefore, changes in renal function as a result of aging will have important pharmacokinetic implications for many drugs.

The renal plasma flow declines by approximately 1% per year and the glomerular filtration rate, corrected for body surface area, decreases at the rate of 1 ml/min/1.73 m^2 per year between the ages of 20 and 90 years. The maximum reabsorptive and maximum excretory capacity of the tubules decline as a function of age.[21,59-62] Thus a gradual decrease in the kidney function occurs with aging.

In a study by Reidenberg et al. involving 23 patients ranging in age from 30 to 90 years significant correlations (inverse) were obtained between age and dose (mg/kg) and plasma concentrations required to produce the same effect[69] Thus, elderly patients required lower doses and lower plasma levels of diazepam than younger patients to achieve the same degree of central nervous system depression. Age-related changes in plasma protein binding cannot account for this effect, since Klotz et al. [33] made the observation that age does not alter the protein binding of diazepam (96.8—98.6%).

Klotz et al.[33] carried out an elegant study to assess the effect of age on the pharmacokinetics of diazepam (0.1 mg/kg given intravenously or orally) in a group of 33 healthy individuals ranging in age from 15 to 82 years (Table 3). These investigators found that the elimination half-life of diazepam increased linearly with age, from 20 hr at age 20 yr to 90 hr at age 80 yr. This increase was a consequence of a very large age-related change (increase) in the volume of distribution (0.5—2.0 1/kg) which predominated, as there was no difference in the plasma clearance values in the two groups (20-30 ml/kg/hr).

The long plasma half-life in the elderly would lengthen the time required to reach steady-state plasma levels, but because of the similar plasma clearance, these levels would be similar in the young and old.[33] The compartmental analysis of the pharmacokinetic data of diazepam did not reveal any changes in the concentration of pharmacologically active drugs in the elderly. Therefore, Klotz and associates concluded that the dosage modification for diazepam in the geriatric patient cannot be solely based on the patients' disposition and elimination characterisitics.[33]

Giles and coworkers also observed that the dose of diazepam required to sedate patients prior to endoscopy was lower in the elderly than in the younger patients.[70]

In another study,[41] diazepam (0.125 mg/kg) was administered intravenously to a group of young healthy subjects (N = 11, ave. age 25 ± 3 yr) and a group of elderly patients (N = 10, ave. age 80 ± 5 yr). No age-related differences

in the elimination half-life of diazepam were observed except in females (54

hr for the young, 66 hr for the elderly). The volume of distribution, which

was larger in females, was significantly increased in the elderly (Table 3).

In a recent study,[71] 9 young (5 females, 21-30 years) and 10 elderly subjects

(5 females, 70-88 years) were given 0.125 mg/kg of diazepam intravenously.

The average elimination half-life in men (32.0 hr) was significantly shorter

than in women (46.2 hr) and plasma clearance in males (33.2 ml/min) was signi-

ficantly larger than in females (18.1 ml/min). The apparent volumes of distri-

bution of diazepam in all males (77.6 1) was not much different than that in

females (76.1 1) but correcting for body weight the values were significantly

lower in young males (1.0 1/kg) as compared to young females (1.28 1/kg). Both

the half-life and volume of distribution in the older subjects (45.1 hr, 1.71

1/kg) were greater than that in the young subjects (35.0 hr, 0.9 1/kg). There

was no conclusive identification of age-dependent differences in the pharamaco-

kinetic parameters due to extensive variation in the values at all ages.

In two groups of subjects aged 17-59 and 60-80 years, given a single oral

dose of diazepam (0.25 mg/kg), peak blood levels of the drug in the younger

group were much higher (140-250 ng/ml) than in the older group (80-90 ng/ml),

but the time taken to reach the peak was the same (60 minutes).[72] The noted[73]

differences in plasma levels of this drug may not be age-related, since large

interindividual variability in the blood levels of diazepam (up to 30-fold) has

been observed in patients receiving the same oral dose .[6,72,74] The absorption

of diazepam even after intramuscular administration is poor and irregular[67,68],

giving rise to plasma levels even lower than after oral administration.[66]

The distribution in cerebrospinal fluid corresponds to the free fraction in

plasma of diazepam (2-3%) and of desmethyldiazepam (1-4%) both after single and

repeated doses.[75] After high doses given for long periods of time, higher levels

of diazepam (8.7% of plasma level) and of desmethyldiazepam (30.9%) were achieved. Any age-related differences in the levels of diazepam or desmethyl-diazepam in the human cerebrospinal fluid have not been described; however, the concentrations of the two compounds achieved in rat brain and cerebrospinal fluid were independent of age.[77]

There is no evidence of a simple correlation between plasma levels of diazepam and desmethyldiazepam and the therapeutic effect.[78] Large variations have been observed between plasma levels of diazepam which are effective after a single dose (about 400 ng/ml) and that after long-term administration (much higher than 400 ng/ml).[72,79-81] Tolerance develops to the therapeutic and side effects of diazepam.[82] The drug also induced its own metabolism after chronic administration.[80,83] Thus, measurement of blood levels of diazepam and des-methyldiazepam is unnecessary except in patients where knowledge of the concentration of the drug could help in clarifying an unexpected reaction.[72,78,81] Plasma level determination can also provide a means of assessing patient compliance and may be especially helpful in cases of suspected diazepam abuse.

It has to be recognized that the metabolites of diazepam contribute significantly to the overall effects of the drug. The pharmacokinetic parameters of the major metabolite, desmethyldiazepam, were found to be modified by age. The half-life of the metabolite in young adults was long (51-120 hr);[79,84] it was even longer (151 hr) in the elderly (4 volunteers 65-85 yr. of age).[85] The clearance was significantly decreased in the elderly, but the volume of distribution was not modified by aging, suggesting the influence of age on the hepatic clearance of the metabolite.

Thus, age-related changes in the formation, accumulation and elimination characteristics of desmethyldiazepam may, at least in part, be responsible for the altered response of diazepam in the elderly.

For the above reasons, diazepam should be given at lower doses, at least initially, in the elderly. Furthermore, a longer duration of residual pharmacological effects should be expected after discontinuation of therapy.

As expected from the altered phsyiology, the renal excretion of drugs,in general,decreases with age. In many cases the elderly patients have higher levels of drugs (e.g. dihydrostreptomycine, tetracyline, sulfamethizole), or increased elimination half-life (e.g. kanamycin, practolol, penicillin, pheno-barbital, acetaminophen, sulfamthizole, digoxin) than in young patients.[25,58,63]

In view of the altered renal function, adjustment of doses of some drugs has to be made to avoid the risk of toxicity in the elderly. Assessment of renal function should be based on creatinine clearance rather than on serum creatinine and blood urea values (the lower renal clearance of creatinine is compensated by lower production of creatinine as a result of smaller muscle mass). Because of the difficulties encountered in obtaining complete 24-hour urines, nomograms have been constructed for determining renal function from serum creatinine con-centrations. These nomograms, which are based upon pharmacokinetic principles and take into account age, sex and body weight, appear to be clinically reli-able.[64]

DIAZEPAM

Diazepam is probably the most widely prescribed drug among the benzodiaze-pines. It is extensively used in the treatment of insomnia, anxiety and as an anticonvulsant. Diazepam is extensively metabolized; less than 2% of an intra-venous dose is excreted unchanged in the urine.[8] The biotransformation products include N-desmethyldiazepam (major), 3-hydroxydiazepam (temazepam), oxazepam and glucuronides.[65,66] Except for the glucuronides, the metabolites are active. Only N-desmethyldiazepam contributes significantly to the overall effect of diazepam.[67]

The frequency of oversedation with diazepam has been noted to increase signi-ficantly between the ages of 40 and 70.[14,68] This may reflect an increased sen-sitivity of the involved receptor site or an increase in the concentration of pharmacologically active drug at the receptor site due to altered pharmacoki-netics as a result of advancing age.

CHLORDIAZEPOXIDE

Chlordiazepoxide was the first of the benzodiazepines to become available for clinical use.[8] Although diazepam has become more popular than chlordiazepoxide, the latter is still prescribed quite extensively.[86]

Chlordiazepoxide is extensively metabolized with less than 1% of an administered dose appearing in urine as parent drug.[86] Among the metabolites of chlordiazepoxide; N-desmethylchlordiazepoxide, demoxepam, desmethyldiazepam and oxazepam have psychopharmacological activity similar to that of the parent drug.[86,87] Therefore, these metabolites must be considered in attempts to interpret the pharmacokinetics and clinical effect of chlordiazepoxide.

After a single intravenous or oral dose desmethylchlordiazepoxide is the major metabolite appearing in plasma. However, after multiple dose administration, both chlordiazepoxide and its pharmacologically active metabolites accumulate at different rates.[81,86,88,89]

The absorption of chlordiazepoxide after oral or intramuscular administration is fairly complete though slow. Considerable variability has been observed in the half-life of chlordiazepoxide (from 6.6 to 28 hr) in normal, healthy volunteers after oral or intravenous dose.[86]

The aging process has an important influence on the pharmacokinetics of chlordiazepoxide. In a series of healthy male volunteers, including 28 young (21-30 years) and 8 old (63-74 years), given 25 mg of chlordiazepoxide orally, the mean elimination half-life in the elderly subjects (18.2 hours) was much longer than in the young individuals (10.1 hours).[27] The absorption in the elderly was slower (ave. half-time of the absorption phase = 19.6 min) than in the young (5.5 min); the total metabolic clearance of the drug in the elderly was also reduced. Tha apparent volume of distribution was significantly larger in the older subjects (0.52 l/kg). There was a parallel reduction in the rate and extent of generation of desmethylchlordiazepoxide in the elderly subjects.[27]

Similar results were obtained by Roberts and associates after intravenous administration of the drug to a group of young and old subjects (24-86 years).[34] The elimination half-life (7-40 hours) and the total clearance (30 ml/min to 10 ml/min) were significantly correlated with age. There was a modest increase in the apparent volume of distribution (0.26 to 0.38 1/kg) with increasing age, but no change in plasma binding (94-97%) of chlordiazepoxide.

No correlation has been found between mean steady-state plasma concentration of chlordiazepoxide (and its metabolities, desmethyldiazepoxide and demoxepam) and clinical anxiolytic effects.[81] On the other hand, Lin and Friedel[89] observed a correlation between the steady-state levels of these metabolites (and not the parent drug) and anxiety reduction. The overall sedative effect at steady-state will depend both on the relative accumulation of the parent drug and its pharmacologically active metabolites as well as the potency of each of the entities.

It is not known whether altered distribution of chlordiazepoxide also leads to an increase in active drug at the receptor site during chronic therapy. Since the elimination half-life is prolonged and total clearance is decreased in the elderly, the steady-state will be reached more slowly and plasma chlordiazepoxide levels will be higher than in the young subjects. Thus, fixed dosage regiments of chlordiazepoxide based upon data obtained in young healthy subjects may result in a slow accumulation of the drug to inappropriately high plasma concentrations in the elderly.

It is difficult to accurately predict the effect of aging on chlordiazepoxide disposition parameters in an individual patient because of considerable inter-individual variability in the magnitude of these parameters and the variable prior history of environmental factors affecting drug disposition. It is recommended that chlordiazepoxide must continue to be used with caution in the elderly.[34]

FLURAZEPAM

Flurazepam hydrochloride has been available in the United States and Canada since 1970 for the treatment of insomnia. Presently, the use of flurazepam in clinical practice is very extensive. Although flurazepam is generally considered to be a safe and effective hypnotic,[8,90,91] recognition of potential unwanted effects of flurazepam and of factors predisposing to toxicity are essential to insure its appropriate use in clinical medicine.

Greenblatt et al.[15,92] reviewed the adverse reactions attributed to flurazepam among 2,542 intensively monitored hospitalized medical patients who received this drug for the treatment of insomnia. Unwanted effects were attributed to the drug in 3.1% of recepients. These effects, which were not serious, included excess central nervous system depression and in all cases the patients recovered spontaneously or following drug discontinuation or reduction of dosage. The frequency of adverse reactions to flurazepam increased significantly as the average daily dose became larger. Toxicity increased with age, progressively from 1.9% among those under 60 years of age to 7.1% among those 80 or over. Although higher doses were associated with a higher frequency of adverse reactions, regardless of age, the effect of dose was most striking in the elderly. Among those 70 or older who received an average daily dose of 30 mg or more, unwanted effects were attributed to flurazepam in 39% of patients. However, at average dialy doses of under 15 mg/day, the unwanted side effects were no more than 2% of cases regardless of age. The findings of the authors suggest that low doses of flurazepam can be safely administered to elderly individuals but that the risk of toxicity increases substantially with large doses.

The mechanism of the apparent enhanced toxicity of high-dose flurazepam in the elderly is not known. The sensitivity of the central nervous system to the depressant effect of flurazepam may be greater in elderly than in young individuals. It is also possible that the pharmacokinetic properties of flurazepam change in relation to age . The frequency of adverse reactions to flurazepam appeared to increase as admission BUN levels became higher. The reasons for this are not entirely clear since renal clearance of either flura- zepam or its metabolic products in their pharmacologically active forms contri- bute very little to their metabolic clearance.[65,93]

Flurazepam is extensively metabolized; even after a large oral dose (90 mg) of flurazapam, peak blood concentrations of the drug were only 10-20 ng/ml.[94] Orally administered flurazepam is so rapidly biotransformed that even during chronic therapy, the intact drug is barely detectable (less than 4 ng/ml) after therapeutic doses (30 mg daily for 2 weeks).[95] Therefore, pharmacokinetic para- meters of only the metabolites have been determined.

The first-pass metabolism of flurazepam, following oral administration, occurs in the small bowel as well as in the liver. The major intestinal meta- bolites were found to be mono- and didesethylflurazepam.[96] The major metabolites in plasma are monodesethyl flurazepam and the hydroxyethyl derivative which possess psychopharmacological activity.[87] The hydroxyethyl metabolite has a short half-life (2 hr)[94,97] while the monodesethyl metabolite has a long eli- mination half-life (51-100 hr).[95] Since significant accumulation of the mono- desethyl metabolite occurs during continuous oral administration of fluraze- pam,[95] it may contribute to the hypnotic and persistent sedative action of flurazepam.[97] The accumulation of active metabolites may explain the delayed peak effectiveness of daily flurazepam therapy.[98]

NITRAZEPAM

Nitrazepam is a widely used, potent, efficacious and relatively safe sleep- inducing agent.[9] Normally at doses of 5-10 mg, it is a safe and satisfactory hypnotic both in healthy volunteers and in elderly psychiatric patients.[99-101] However, a single dose of 5 mg of the drug given to middle-aged policemen has been reported to interefere with their driving skill,[101] and the same dose given to geriatric patients caused confusion and disorientation.[102] Increased sensitivity to nitrazepam in old age at a dose of 10 mg was shown by Castleden and associates.[103] During chronic use, especially in old patients, nitrazepam given at bed time may produce muscle relaxation, sedation, drowsiness and impairment of certain skills which persist during the daytime. Kangas et al.,[35] reported that aged patients were more sensitive to the sedative effect of nitrazepam than the young volunteers. The pharmacodynamic effects of nitrazepam appear to be dependent on the dose and on the age of the subjects.

A survey involving more than 2000 hospitalized medical patients was carried out to assess the potential hazard of nitrazepam therapy of insomnia.[16] Unwanted central nervous system depression (drowsiness and/or hangover) attributed to nitrazepam was substantially more frequent among the elderly, particularly in patients aged 70 years or more. The effect of age on the reported rate of unwanted CNS depression was most striking at high doses. Among patients aged 80 years or over whose daily dose average 10 mg or more, 55% experienced unwanted CNS depression. These findings suggest that there is little reason to exceed a 5 mg dose of nitrazepam for most patients particularly the elderly.[16]

Castleden et al.[103] found similar plasma concentrations of nitrazepam in both young (mean age 25 yr) and elderly (N = 10, mean age 75 yr) apparently healthy subjects given 10 mg of the drug orally. The elimination half-life of nitrazepam (32.8 hr) and the apparent volume of distribution (2.8 l/kg) were almost identical in the two groups. Therefore, the increased effect of nitrazepam on psychomotor performance in the elderly was attributed to the increased sensitivity of the aging brain to the action of the drug without and age-related change in pharmacokinetics.

On the other hand, Kangas et al.[35] found a clear increase in the plasma half-life (ave. 40.4 hr) of nitrazepam after a single 5 mg oral dose in a group of geriatric patients (Group 1, ave. age 77 yr) who were partly or totally bedridden when compared to a group of young volunteers (ave. age 24 yr). These patients differed from the apparently healthy group of elderly subjects in the study by Castleden and coworkers.[103] It is possible that the impairment of the circulation in totally bedridden patients may change the pharmacokinetic profile of drugs. Hence, the immobility of patients, their disease, and other medications may be determinants of the pharmacokinetic differences of nitrazepam observed between the young and the elderly.[35]

Nevertheless, after cessation of prolonged drug treatment, the elimination half-life of nitrazepam (39.8 hr) in elderly patients (Group 2, mean age = 81 yr) who were non-debilitated was much higher than that in young volunteers (mean age = 25 yr., ave. half-life = 24.2).[35] Peak plasma concentrations of nitrazepam in sick geriatric patients were about one-half of those in the young volunteers after the single dose; this was explained by decreased absorption in the elderly. After prolonged administration, the steady-state levels of nitrazepam in the elderly patients (Group 2) were lower and were achieved more slowly (7.5 days vs. 3.5 days) than in the young volunteers.

The apparent volume of distribution in the elderly was significantly higher (4.8 l/kg) than the younger subjects (2.4 l/kg). Nitrazepam, being lipophilic, will accumulate in the relatively larger lipid body compartment in the elderly accounting for the apparent increase in the volume of distribution.[35] Antipyrine by comparison, which is distributed throughout total body water, has a decreased apparent volume of distribution in the elderly.[25]

The apparent volume of distribution may be the most important factor in modification of the pharmacokinetic and pharmacodynamic properties of nitrazepam. In the aged subjects with higher volume of distribution at steady-state, a greater amount of the administered dose will be present in the tissue compartment, and presumably at receptor sites in the central nervous system. Because nitrazepam is eliminated from the cerebral spinal fluid even more slowly than from plasma,[105] the increased frequency of central side effects and increased sensitivity to nitrazepam in the elderly[102,103] could be due to an altered distribution pattern. It is not known whether the binding of nitrazepam to plasma proteins (85-88%) is modified by age.

Nitrazepam is extensively metabolized; less than 1% is excreted unchanged in the urine.[106] A large interindividual variation was observed in the urinary elimination of the total drug (17-99% in 7 days; 57% as conjugates).[106] Fecal elimination accounts for only a few percent of the administered dose.[107] It appears that a large fraction of the drug binds to tissues in a "deep compartment" from which it is slowly eliminated.[106]

The metabolic pathways of nitrazepam have not been fully determined; the drug is metabolized in part by nitro-reduction to the amine (7-aminonitrazepam) followed by acetylation to 7-acetamidonitrazepam.[106,108a] The acetylation step has been shown to be under the control of genetric polymorphism.[109a] These metabolites are excreted as such and as glucuronides.[106] Unlike diazepam, nitrazepam does not induce or inhibit its own disposition during long-term treatment.[35]

OXAZEPAM

Oxazepam, one of the first benzodiazepines introduced into clinical use, is an effective and safe drug.[108b] It has been reported that side effects with oxazepam are fewer than with diazepam and chlordiazepoxide even in the elderly.[109b,110]

Oxazepam is rapidly absorbed and is one of the fastest acting benzodiazepine.[109b,111] Oxazepam has a much shorter half-life than other benzodiazepines, hence there is less chance of accumulation of the drug during chronic therapy.[8] Since oxazepam does not have active metabolites, the clinical response is consistent and predictable, and it has a low potential for drug interaction.[112]

The pharmacokinetic parameters of oxazepam are not affected by age. In 8 young (ave. age 25 yr) and 8 older subjects (ave. age 54 yr), the elimination half-life (5.1 vs. 5.6 hr) , the apparent volume of distribution (48 1 vs. 61 1) and the urinary excretion of the total drug (51 vs. 55%, mostly as glucuronide) were not significantly different. The binding to plasma (86.7 vs 89.3%) or the blood to plasma ratio of oxazepam (1.04 vs 0.96) was also the same in the two groups.[111,113]

The lack of effect of age on the disposition of oxazepam may be due to its short half-life and its exclusive route of metabolism viz. glucuronidation,[114] which is apparently not influenced by age.

Because of the above reasons and its wide margin of safety, oxazepam is es-pecially suitable for use in the elderly.[109b,110]

LORAZEPAM

Lorazepam is a newer benzodiazepine. It has been found to be superior to pentobarbital as a surgical premedicant in that lorazepam provides greater se-dation, lack of recall and greater antianxiety effect than does pentobarbital (128 pt., 18-65 yr).[115]

Lorazepam, like oxazepam is extensively metabolized by glucuronidation;[116-119] however, the elimination half-life of lorazepam is much longer than that of oxazepam. After an oral dose (2 mg, 8 healthy young males), the drug was ab-sorbed with an apparent first-order half-time of 15 minutes, following a lag time of 30 min.[118] The peak plasma levels were obtained at about 2 hours (cor-responding to the time at which clinical effects appear to be maximal). The apparent elimination half-life of lorazepam was about 12 hr. The major meta-bolite, the glucuronide, was formed rapidly. About 75% of the dose of lorazepam was excreted in the urine as the glucuronide in 5 days.[118] The glucuronide was eliminated with a half-life of 15.3 hr.[119] The binding of the glucuronide to plasma proteints (65%)[118] was much lower than the binding of lorazepam (93.2% at therapeutic conditions).[120] The true course of clinical effects paralleled plasma concentrations of free lorazepam rather than lorazepam glucuronide.

The pharmacokinetic parameters of lorazepam have been reported to be somewhat modified by age. In 15 healthy young subjects given 1.5 to 30 mg of lorazepam intravenously, the volume of distribution in the elderly group (0.99 1/kg) was slightly but significantly smaller than in the young group (1.11 1/kg), suggesting less extensive drug distribution in the elderly.[29] Although the values of elimination half-life of the drug in the elderly (15.9 hr) did not differ significantly from those in the young group (14.1 hr), the total clearance in the elderly (0.77 ml/min/kg) was significantly lower than in the young subjects (0.99 ml/min/kg).[29] The kinetic data varied considerably among individuals in both age groups.

In another study involving 11 apparently healthy, normal male individuals ranging in age from 15 to 73 years, given 2 mg of lorazepam intravenously, no statistically significant age-dependent relationships in the drug's pharmacokinetic parameters were observed.[40] This included measurements of plasma half-life (ave. = 21.7 hr), plasma clearance (0.75 1/min/kg) and apparent volume of distribution (1.28 1/kg). These data indicate that the disposition of lorazepam after a single small dose, is not affected by the aging process. This lack of effect upon drug metabolism suggests that the glucuronidation pathway of biotransformation may be more resistant to the effect of the biochemical and physiological changes associated with aging than are the oxidative processes.

LITHIUM

The efficacy of lithium, either alone or in combination with tricyclic antidepressants, in the treatment of manic-depressive illness is well-establish-ed.[18-20] Lithium in combination with antipsychotic drugs has been effective in patients who have previously failed other treatments.[122]

Lithium is one drug for which a knowledge of pharmacokinetics is not only useful in the clinical situation, but also must now be considered essential for optimum therapy, both in terms of efficacy and safety. The dose requirement between individuals varies within very wide limits (8-80 mmol Li/day). The therapeutic range of lithium concentration in the plasma is narrow, and the levels vary appreciately in the course of 24 hours in relation to the intake of tablets. For this reason, recommendations were made to adjust the dosage to achieve a serum lithium concentration around 1.0 mmole/l. A standardized 12 hour serum lithium concentration has been defined as the concentration of lith-ium in the serum from a blood sample drawn in the morning exactly 12 hours after the last dose of lithium in a patient who has been taking the daily lithium in two or more divided doses and who has been taking all of the prescribed dose at the scheduled hours during the past 48 hours.[19,123] This standardized procedure has been used to establish the therapeutic range and to determine whether a patient is within the range. When severe, intolerable side effects are seen at this serum concentration range, they can be controlled by rapid reduction of the dose. It may be noted that steady-state levels of lithium in serum and tissues are achieved after 5 to 7 days of daily doses of the drug.[121]

Serum levels of lithium should not be used as the only therapeutic index, es-pecially in the elderly; one should regard clinical status as the most important indicator of therapeutic efficacy and of toxicity.

When administered orally as a dilute solution of lithium chloride, it is ra-pidly and completely absorbed. However, when lithium is administered in the form of tablets, the absorption is variable. After its rapid absorption, lith-ium is distributed at a somewhat slower rate (6-10 hours for complete distri-bution). The elimination half-life of lithium in patients with normal renal function varies interindividually between 7 and 24 hours during the daytime; it is longer during the night time (night/day ration of half-life = 1.15-2.48). The renal clearance of lithium in subjects with normal renal function was found to be 10-40 ml/min.[124] In another study, the elimination half-life in 12 schizo-phrenic patients (age 20-62 years, only 2 above 50) ranged from 19.3 to 41.3 hours (ave. = 28.9 hours). A significant correlation was found between the elimination half-life and renal creatinine clearance;[125] but in this small group of patients, a correlation between elimination half-life and age was not apparent.

The lithium ion is non-protein bound and is fairly evenly distributed in the body except in tissues such as white matter of the brain, the bones, and the thyroid gland in which the concentrations are about twice those in the serum.[123] The apparent distribution volume in young subjects was found to be 1.2 1/kg while in the older population, it was 0.9 1/kg.[124]

Since lithium is excreted almost entirely by the kidneys, one would expect a decreased clearance of lithium in the elderly (due to decreased endogeneous creatinine clearance). The elimination of lithium from the kidneys is also related to the amount of sodium intake. Sodium depleting agents such as diuretics (often taken by the elderly patients) may result in the retention of lithium. Thiazide diuretics may decrease renal clearance of lithium by 25% to 50%.[126] On the other hand, decreased levels of lithium can result from high salt or sodium bicarbonate intake which might be the case in the elderly. High intercellular levels may occur due to accumulation in the elderly. Lithium poisoning is an extremely dangerous condition leading to permanent neurological damage or even death.[121] Consequently, the dose of lithium in the elderly (both the starting as well as maintenance) should be carefully adjusted downwards and plasma levels should be monitored.

Caution should be exercized if lithium is used with other psychotrophic drugs since serious side effects could result in the elderly. For example, lithium with tricyclic antidepressants can cause seizure, delirium and low blood pressure (even with low dosages of the tricyclic antidepressants in some patients). Combination of lithium with diazepam or oxazepam may increase central nervous system depression in elderly patients who are particularly sensitive.[121]

POSSIBLE MECHANISMS FOR INCREASED RESPONSE OF BENZODIAZEPINES IN THE ELDERLY

The exact neuronal site and molecular mechanism of action of benzodiazepines is unknown. Recently, a benzodiazepine receptor has been identified in the rodent central nervous system[127-131] and in human brain.[132,133] Benzodiazepines bind to this cell surface receptor in the human brain in a selective and stereospecific fashion. A 24-fold difference was found in the areas of highest (cerebral cortex) and the lowest (brain stem) specific binding for diazepam (tritium labelled). The therapeutic and pharmacological potency of benzodiaze-pines closely parallels the affinity to the binding site. This binding site in human brain may represent the site of central action of benzodiazepines.[132]

Increased sensitivity of benzodiazepines in the elderly may be due to (1) in-creased intrinsic sensitivity of the receptor in the brain, (2) increased levels of drug (and active metabolites) at this receptor. The concentration of the active agent at the receptor could increase as a result of (a) increased per-meability of the central nervous system, (b) increase in the ratio of the total number of receptors to the total weight of the brain (decrease of drug-binding-tissue) and (c) increased levels of free drug (and active metabolites) at the re-ceptor as a result of pharmacokinetic changes inside and outside the central nervous system, and (3) alteration in the levels of neurochemicals which may be involved in the mediation of benzodiazepine action.

Not much is known about the age-related changes that occur in the receptor sensitivity in the brain except that the aging human brain becomes more sensi-tive to many drugs.[25,46,69,103,134]

Age-related changes in the permeability of central nervous system or the integrity of the blood-brain-barrier are not known.

It has been shown that the brain protein synthesis (lysine incorporation into protein in the various areas of the brain) declines progressively with increasing age.[135] In man, brain weight decreases linearly with age[136,137] with the largest reduction occurring after the sixth or seventh postnatal decade.[137,138] Some of the brain atrophy seen during senescence may be caused by a loss of nerve cells in the central nervous system.[139,140] Thus, there may be a reduction in the total drug-binding tissue in the brain and a concomitant increase in the level of free drug at the receptor site (assuming no age-related change in the number of recep-tor sites).

There is another mechanism by which the concentration of free drug can increase in the brain: brain and spinal cord water and lipids decrease with old age.[141-143] Thus, a reduction in the distribution volume will increase the concentration of the free drug in the brain.

The pharmacokinetic changes which have been demonstrated to occur with aging are described for a number of benzodiazepines (see earlier). These changes may result in an increase of free level of the drug (or active metabolites) in the brain.

A host of neurotransmitter systems, including acetylcholine, catecholamines, serotonin, γ-aminobutyric acid (GABA) and glycine have been proposed to partici- pate in the anxiolytic, myorelaxant and anticonvulsant action of the benzodia- zepines.[144,145]

A theory has been postulated that GABA transmission is the focal point in the mode of action of benzodiazepines. The interaction between the benzodiazepines and the allosteric protein modulator of GABA recognition sites may be relevant to explain the in vivo action of the benzodiazepines on GABA transmission. The rank order of potency for a small number of benzodiazepines to compete with the protein modulator is similar to that which causes a relief of anxiety.[144] Diaze- pam alters the cyclic GMP content of cerebellar cortex by acting through the γ-aminobutyric acid (GABA) receptor, pssibly by increasing the affinity of the receptor for GABA[146]. It is unknown if age-related changes occur in the levels of cyclic GMP, GABA or response of GABA-receptor to GABA.

Brain tissue has rather high activities of adenylate cyclase and phosphodi- esterases and possesses a relatively high concentration of cyclic GMP. Psychotro- phic drugs, including some benzodiazepines, have been shown to interfere with cyclic-GMP generating and degrading systems.[148.149] It is not known whether the activity of these enzymes within the brain is modified as a result of aging and increase in the sensitivity of the aging brain to psychotrophic drugs has any correlation with changes in the activity of enzymes or level of cyclic GMP.

TABLE 3

PHARMACOKINETIC PARAMETERS

Drug/Dose	Subjects	Age (yrs)	Pharmacokinetic Parameters	Ref.
DIAZEPAM 0.1 mg/kg i.v. or p.o.	33V	15-82	$t_{1/2}$ increased linearly with age, from 20 hr at 20 yr to 90 hr at 80 yr; Cp higher in young than in elderly; no change in plasma Cl	33
0.125 mg/kg i.v.	11V	(25)	Male, $t_{1/2}$ = 42 hr; Vd = 1.0 l/kg Female, $t_{1/2}$ = 66 hr; Vd = 1.8 l/kg	41
	10P	(80)	Male, $t_{1/2}$ = 45 hr; Vd = 1.8 l/kg Female, $t_{1/2}$ = 54 hr; Vd = 2.4 l/kg	
0.125 mg/kg i.v.	9V	21-30 (26)	$t_{1/2}$ = 35 hr; Vd = 0.9 l/kg Cl = 26.9 ml/min	71
	10V	70-88 (82)	$t_{1/2}$ = 45 hr; Vd = 1.7 l/kg Cl = 32.4 ml/min	
2-30 mg, p.o. daily for 6 weeks	50P	24-72	Cp of diazepam and desmethyldiazepam were inversely related to age	150
5-10 mg, iv.	16V	26-37	Male, $t_{1/2}$ = 39 hr; Vd = 1.16 l/kg Cl = 0.37 ml/min/kg Female, $t_{1/2}$ = 44 hr; Vd = 1.69 l/kg Cl = 0.47 ml/min/kg	151
5-10 mg, i.v.	14V	61-84	Male, $t_{1/2}$ = 94; hr; Vd = 1.70 l/kg; Cl = 0.24 ml/min/kg Female, $t_{1/2}$ = 86 hr; Vd = 2.97 l/kg; Cl = 0.43 ml/min/kg	151
CHLORDIAZEPOXIDE 25 mg, p.o.	28V	21-30 (25)	$t_{1/2}(\alpha)$ = 5.5 min; Cp(peak) = 0.86 ug/ml; $t_{1/2}$ = 10.1 hr; Vd = 0.42 l/kg; Cl = 46.3 ml/min	27
	8V	63-74 (67)	$t_{1/2}(\alpha)$ = 19.6 min; Cp(peak) = 0.69 ug/ml; $t_{1/2}$ = 18.2 hr; Vd = 0.52 l/kg Cl = 26.6 ml/min	
0.6 mg/kg i.v.	20V	24-86	$t_{1/2}$ (7-40 hr) correlated with age	34
OXAZEPAM 45 mg, p.o.	8V	14-30 (25)	$t_{1/2}$ = 5.1 hr; Vd = 48 l	111 113
	8V	45-84 (54)	$t_{1/2}$ = 5.6 hr; Vd = 61 l	
NITRAZEPAM 5 mg p.o.	25V	18-38	$t_{1/2}$ = 28.9 hr; Vd = 2.4 l/kg $Cl_{(total)}$= 4.1 l/hr; Cp(max) = 39.9 ng/ml	35
	20P	66-89 (77)	$t_{1/2}$ = 40.4 hr; Vd = 4.8 l/kg $Cl_{(total)}$ = 4.7 l/hr; Cp(max) = 21.8 ng/ml	
5 mg, p.o. daily for 2 weeks	11V	21-33 (25)	$t_{1/2}$ = 24.2 hr; Cp (steady-state) = 57 ng/ml	35
	10V	73-94 (81)	$t_{1/2}$ = 39.8 hr; Cp (steady-state) = 45 ng/ml	

Drug/Dose	Subjects	Age (yr)	Pharmacokinetic Parameters	Ref.
NITRAZEPAM (con't)				
10 mg, p.o.	10V	(25)	$t_{1/2}$ = 32.5 hr; Vd = 2.9 1/kg (no correlation with age)	103
	10V	(75)	$t_{1/2}$ = 33.0 hr; Vd = 2.7 1/kg	
LORAZEPAM	6V	22-34	$t_{1/2}(\alpha)$ = 21 min; Vd = 0.9 1/kg	
4 mg, i.m.		(27)	$t_{1/2}$ = 13.6 hr; Cl = 58.2 ml/min	119
2 mg, i.v.	11V	15-73	$t_{1/2}$ = 21.7 hr; Vd = 1.28 1/kg Cl = 0.7 ml/min/kg (no change with age)	40
1.5-3 mg, i.v.	16V	19-38	$t_{1/2}(\alpha)$ = 2.6 min; Vd = 0.99 1/kg	29
		(27)	$t_{1/2}$ = 14.1 hr, Cl = 0.99 ml/min/kg	
	16V	60-84	$t_{1/2}(\alpha)$ = 3.1 min; Vd = 1.11 1/kg	
		(70)	$t_{1/2}$ = 15.9 hr; Cl = 0.77 ml/min/kg	
1.5-3 mg, i.m.	11V	60-76	$t_{1/2}(\alpha)$ = 15.6 min	29
			$t_{1/2}$ = 17.7 hr	
1.5-3 mg, p.o.	11V	60-76	$t_{1/2}(\alpha)$ = 10.9 min	29
			$t_{1/2}$ = 17.2 hr	
LITHIUM	13V		$t_{1/2}$ = 7-24 hr; Cl = 10-40 ml/min	124
24 mmole p.o.			No correlation with age; Vd = 1.2 1/kg in young, Vd = 0.9 1/kg in old	123
		20-62	$t_{1/2}$ = 28.9 hr (19.3-41.3)	125
		(26)	No correlation with age	

( ) = average; V = volunteers, P= patients; $t_{1/2}$ = plasma elimination half-life; $t_{1/2}(\alpha)$ = half-life of distribution; Vd = apparent volume of distribution; Cl = clearance, Cp = plasma level

SUMMARY

Benzodiazepines are extensively prescribed for the elderly mostly for insomnia and anxiety. Although these drugs possess a wide margin of therapeutic safety, their use (especially in the elderly) is not without a considerable incidence of side effects. The efficacy of lithium in the treatment of psychotic and manic-depressive illness is well established. The potential for toxicity of lithium in the elderly is fairly high. Recognition of potential unwanted effects of these drugs and of factors predisposing the toxicity are important to insure appropriate use in clinical medicine.

Aging is generally associated with many physiological and biochemical changes which affect tissue reactivity, sensitivity and tolerance to drugs by modifica-

tions of the drug action at the molecular level. The altered response to various drugs in the elderly could be due to age-related modification of the site(s)
of action and/or modification of the pharmacokinetic profile of the drug resulting in altered level of free drug at its site(s) of action.

Age-related changes have been reported to occur in the pharmacokinetic parameters of drugs. Among the benzodiazepines, the rate but not the extent of absorption of chlordiazepoxide and lorazepam is decreased in the elderly. The
apparent volume of distribution in the elderly is larger than in young subjects
for diazepam, oxazepam, chlordiazepoxide, nitrazepam and lorazepam. The elimination half-life from plasma is increased in the case of diazepam, chlordiazepoxide, nitrazepam and lorazepam, but not for oxazepam. In general, lower plasma
levels are reached in the elderly after   single oral doses of benzodiazepines.
However, after chronic dosing, steady-state levels are higher and are achieved
more slowly when compared to the young subjects. The renal clearance of drugs
is lower in the elderly. Accumulation of drug and active metabolites after
chronic dosing is more likely to occur with chlordiazepoxide, diazepam, flurazepam and nitrazepam. It has been suggested that the aging brain becomes more
sensitive to the depressant action of diazepam, chlordiazepoxide and nitrazepam.

Based upon pharmacokinetic data and the reported increase in the sensitivity
of the central nervous system in the elderly, the doses of diazepam, chlordiazepoxide, flurazepam and nitrazepam should be decreased in the elderly. Among the
benzodiazepines, oxazepam and flurazepam appear to be "safer" drugs for use in
the elderly.

Lithium is excreted almost entirely by the kidneys and its elimination is
also related to the amount of sodium intake. Diuretics may decrease renal clearance of lithium. High intercellular levels may occur due to accumulation in the
elderly. Since lithium has a narrow therapeutic range and lithium poisoning is
an extremely dangerous condition leading to permanent neurological damage or
even death, the dose of lithium in the elderly (both the starting as well as

58

maintenance) should be carefully adjusted downward and plasma levels should be monitored. Furthermore, caution should be exercized if lithium is used with other psychotropic drugs such as tricyclic antidepressants and benzodiazepines, since serious side effects could result with the combination in the elderly.

ACKNOWLEDGEMENT

The author would like to thank Mr. David Masel, Ms. Barbara Kell and Ms. Suzanne Raymund for their help in preparing the manuscript.

REFERENCES

1. Fottrell, E., Sheikh, M., Kothari, R. and Sayed, I. (1976) Lancet, 1, 81.
2. Chapman, S.S. (1976) Med. J. Aust., 2, 62.
3. Bergman, U., Dahlstrom, M., Gunnarsson, C. and Westerholm, B. (1979) Eur. J. Clin. Pharmacol., 15, 249.
4. Learoyd, B.M. (1972) Med. J. Aust., 1, 1131.
5. Achong, M.R., Bayne, J.R.D., Gerson, L.W. and Golshani, S. (1978) Can. Med. J., 118, 1503.
6. Garattini, S., Marcucci, F., Morselli, P.L. and Mussini, E. (1973) In Biological Effects of Drugs in Relation to Their Plasma Concentrations, Davies, D.S. and Pritchard, B.N.C. ed., MacMillan, London, pp. 211-225.
7. Garattini, S., Marcucci, G., Morselli, P.L. and Mussini, E. (1975) In Handbook of Experimental Pharmacology, Vol. 28, Davies, D.S. and Pritchard, B.N.C. ed., Springer-Verlag, New York, pp. 113-119.
8. Greenblatt, D.J. and Shader, R.I. (1974) Benzodiazepines in Clinical Practice, Raven Press, New York.
9. Greenblatt, D.J. and Shader, R.I. (1974) N. Engl. J. Med., 291, 1011.
10. Greenblatt, D.J. and Shader, R.I. (1974) N. Engl. J. Med., 291, 1239.
11. Seller, E.M. (1978) Cancer Med. Assoc. J., 118, 1533.
12. Dawson-Butterworth, K. (1970) J. Amer. Geriat. Soc., 18, 297.
13. Learoyd, B.M. (1974) Med. J. Aust., 1, 475.
14. Boston Collaborative Surveillance Drug Program (1973) N. Engl. J. Med., 288, 277.
15. Greenblatt, D.J., Allen, M.D., Noel, J. and Shader, R.I. (1977) Clin. Pharmacol. Ther., 21, 355.
16. Greenblatt, D.J. and Allen, M.D. (1978) Brit. J. Clin. Pharmacol., 5, 407.
17. Miller, R.R. and Greenblatt, D.J. (1976) Drug Effects in Hospitalized Patients: Experiences of the Boston Collaborative Drug Surveillance Program 1966-75, Wiley, N.Y.
18. Shou, M., Juel-Nielsen, N., Stromgren, E. and Voldby, H. (1954) J. Neurolog. Neurosurg. Psychiat., 17, 250.
19. Amdisen, A. (1977) Clin. Pharmacokin., 2, 73.
20. Prien, P.F. (1978) Clin. Neuro. Pharmacol., 3, 113.
21. Bender, A.D. (1965) J. Amer. Geriat. Soc., 13, 192.
22. Sherlock, S., Bearn, A.G., Billing, B.H. and Paterson, J.C.S. (1950) J. Lab. Clin. Med., 35, 923.
23. Brandfonbrener, M., Landowne, M. and Shock, N.W. (1955) Circulation, 12, 557.

24. Warren, P.M., Pepperman, M.A. and Montgomery, R.D. (1978) Lancet, 2, 849.
25. Crooks, J., O'Malley, K. and Stevenson, I.H. (1976) Clin. Pharmacokinet., 1, 280.
26. Israili, Z.H. (1979) Aging (in press).
27. Shader, R.I., Greenblatt, D.J., Harmatz, J.S., Franke, K. and Koch-Weser, J. (1977) J. Clin. Pharmacol., 17, 709.
28. Cusack, B., Horgan, J., Kelley, J.G., Lavan, J., Noel, J. and O'Malley, K. (1978) Brit. J. Clin. Pharmacol., 6, 439P.
29. Greenblatt, D.J., Allen, M.D., Locniskar, A., Harmatz, J.S. and Shader, R.I. (1979) Clin. Pharmacol. Ther. 26, 103.
30. Shader, R.I., Georgotas, A., Greenblatt, D.J., Harmatz, J.S. and Allen, M.D. (1978) Clin. Pharmacol. Ther., 24, 308.
31. Edelman, I.S. and Leibman, J. (1959) Am. J. Med., 27, 256.
32. Novak, L.P. (1972) J. Gerontol., 27, 438.
33. Klotz, U., Avant, G.R., Hoyumpa, A., Schenker, S. and Wilkinson, G.R. (1975) J. Clin. Invest., 55, 347.
34. Roberts, R.K., Wilkinson, G.R., Branch, R.A. and Schenker, S. (1978) Gastro-enterology, 75, 479.
35. Kangas, L., Iisalo, E., Kanto, J., Lehtinen, V., Pynnonen, S., Ruikka, I., Salminen, J., Sillapaa, M. and Syvalahti, E. (1979) Eur. J. Clin. Pharma-col., 15, 163.
36. O'Malley, K., Crooks, J., Duke, E. and Stevenson, I.H. (1971) Brit. Med. J., 3, 607.
37. Simon, C., Malerczyk, V., Muller, U. and Muller, G. (1972) Deutsch. Med. Worchenschr., 97, 1999.
38. Triggs, E.J., Nation, R.L., Long, A. and Ashley, J.J. (1975) Eur. J. Clin. Pharmacol., 8, 55.
39. Hewick, D.S., Moreland, T.A., Shepherd, A.M.M. and Stevenson, I.H. (1975) Brit. Med. J., 2, 189.
40. Kraus, J.W., Desmond, P.V., Marshall, J.P., Johnson, R.F., Schenker, S. and Wilkinson, G.R. (1978) Clin. Pharmacol. Ther., 24, 411.
41. McLeod, S.M., Giles, H.G., Bengert, B., Liu, F. and Sellers, E.M. (1979) Clin. Res., 25, 676A.
42. Woodford-Williams, E., Alvares, A.S., Webster, D., Landless, B. and Dixon, M.P. (1964) Gerontologia, 10, 86.
43. Greenblatt, D.J. (1979) J. Am. Geriat. Soc., 27, 20.
44. Houghton, G.W., Richens, A. and Leighton, M. (1975) Brit. J. Clin. Pharma-col., 2, 251.
45. Hayes, M.J., Langman, M.J.S. and Short, A.H. (1975) Brit. J. Clin. Pharma-col., 2, 73.
46. Mather, L.E., Tucker, G.T., Pslug, A.E., Lindop, J. and Wilkerson, C. (1975) Clin. Pharmacol. Ther., 17, 21.
47. Wallace, S., Whiting, B. and Runcie, J. (1976) Brit. J. Clin. Pharmacol., 3, 327.
48. Bender, A.D., Post, A., Meier, J.P., Higson, J.E. and Reichard, G. (1975) J. Pharm. Sci., 64, 1711.
49. Chan, K., Kendall, M.J., Mitchard, M. and Wells, W.D.E. (1975) Brit. J. Clin. Pharmacol., 2, 297.
50. Ehrnebo, M., Agurell, S., Boreus, L.O., Gordon, E. and Lonrotti, U. (1974) Clin. Pharmacol. Ther., 16, 424.
51. Castleden, C.M. and George, C.F. (1979) Brit. J. Clin. Pharmacol., 7, 49.
52. Vestal, R.E., Wood, A.J.J., Branch, R.A., Shand, D.G. and Wilkinson, G.R. (1979) Clin. Pharmacol. Ther., 26, 8.
53. Wood, A.J.J., Vestal, R.E., Wilkinson, G.R., Branch, R.A. and Shand, D.G. (1979) Clin. Pharmacol. Ther., 26, 16.
54. Kato, R., Vassanelli, P., Frontino, G. and Chiesara, E. (1964) Biochem. Pharmacol., 13, 1037.
55. Kato, R. and Takanka, A. (1968) J. Biochem., (Tokyo), 63, 406.

56. Kato, R. and Takanka, A. (1968) Jap. J. Pharmacol., 18, 387.
57. Triggs, E.J. and Nation, R.L. (1975) J. Pharmacokinet. Biopharm., 3, 387.
58. Richey, D.P. and Bender, A.D. (1977) Ann. Rev. Pharmacol. Toxicol., 17, 49.
59. Davies, D.F. and Shock, N.W. (1950) J. Clin. Invest., 29, 496.
60. Malholm-Hansen, J., Kampmann, J. and Laursen, H. (1970) Lancet, 1, 1170.
61. Rowe, J.W., Andres, R., Tobin, J.D., Norris, A.H. and Shock, N.W. (1976)
    Ann. Intern. Med., 84, 567.
62. Gaul, M.H. and Cockcroft, D.W. (1975) Lancet, 2, 613.
63. Briant, R.H., Dorrington, R.W., Cleal, J. and Williams, F.M. (1976) J.
    Amer. Geriat. Soc., 24, 359.
64. Bjornsson, J.D. (1979) Clin. Pharmacokin., 4, 200.
65. Schwartz, M.A. and Postma, E. (1970) J. Pharm. Sci., 59, 1800.
66. Hillestad, L., Hansen, T., Melsom, H. and Drivenes, A. (1974) Clin. Pharma-
    col. Ther., 16, 479.
67. Mandelli, M., Tognoni, G. and Garattini, S. (1978) Clin. Pharmacokin., 3,
    72.
68. Greenblatt, D.J. (1976) Antianxiety agents, Miller, R.R. and Greenblatt,
    D.J., ed., New York, pp. 193-203.
69. Reidenberg, M.M., Levy, M., Warner, H., Coutinho, C.B., Schwartz, M.A.,
    Yu, G. and Cheripko, J. (1978) Clin. Pharmacol. Ther., 23, 371.
70. Giles, H.G., McLeod, S.M., Wright, J.R. and Sellers, E.M. (1978) Can. Med.
    Assoc. J., 118, 513.
71. MacLeod, S.M., Giles, H.G., Bengert, B., Liu, F.F. and Sellers, E.M. (1979)
    J. Clin. Pharmacol., 19, 15.
72. Garattini, S., Mussini, E. and Randall, L.O. (1973) Benzodiazepines, Mario
    Negri Inst. Monograph, Raven Press, New York.
73. Rutherford, D.M., Okoko, A. and Tyrer, P.J. (1978) Brit. J. Clin. Pharma-
    col., 6, 69.
74. Gamble, J.A.S., Dundee, J.W. and Assaf, R.A.E. (1975) Anaesthesia, 30, 149.
75. Kanto, J., Kangas, L. and Siirtola, T. (1975) Acta Pharmacol. Toxicol.,
    36, 328.
76. Hendel, J. (1975) Acta Pharmacol. Toxicol., 37, 17.
77. Klotz, U. (1979) Naunyn-Schmiedeberg's Arch. Pharmacol., 307, 167.
78. Tansella, M., Zimmermann, C.H., Tansella, L., Ferrario, L., Preziati, L.,
    Tognoni, G. and Lader, M. (1978) Pharmakopsychiatrie, in press.
79. Tansella, M., Siciliani, O., Burti, L., Schiavon, M., Zimmermann, T.,
    Gerna, M., Tognoni, G. and Morselli, P. L. (1975) Psychopharmacologia, Ber-
    lin, 41, 81.
80. Kanto, J., Iisalo, E., Lehtinen, V. and Salminen, J. (1974) Psychopharma-
    cologia (Berl.), 36, 123.
81. Bond, A.J., Hailey, D.M. and Lader, M.H. (1977) Brit. J. Clin. Pharmacol.,
    4, 51.
82. Kales, A., Bixler, E. O., Tan, T.-L. (1974) J. Amer. Med. Assoc., 337,
    513.
83. Sellmann, R., Kanto, J., Raiijola, E. and Pekkarinen, A. (1975) Acta Phar-
    macol. Toxicol., 37, 345.
84. Tognoni, G., Gomeni, R., DeMaio, D., Alberti, G.G., Franciosi, P. and
    Schieghi, G. (1975) Brit. J. Clin. Pharmacol., 2, 227.
85. Klotz, U. and Muller-Seydlitz, P. (1979) Brit. J. Clin. Pharmacol., 7, 119.
86. Greenblatt, D.J., Shader, R.I., MacLeod, S.M. and Sellers, E.M. (1978)
    Clin. Pharmacokin., 3, 381.
87. Randall, L.O. and Kappell, B. (1973) in The Benzodiazepines, Garattini, E.,
    Mussini, E. and Randall, L.O., ed., Raven Press, New York, pp. 27-51.
88. Boxenbaum, H.G., Geitner, K.A., Jack, M.L., Dixon, W.R. and Kaplan, S.A.
    (1977) J. Pharmacokin. Biopharmaceut., 5, 25.
89. Lin, K.-M. and Friedel, R.O. (1978) Am. J. Psychiatry, in press.
90. Greenblatt, D.J., Shader, R.I. and Koch-Weser, J. (1975) Clin. Pharmacol.
    Ther., 17, 1.

91. Greenblatt, D.J., Shader, R.I. and Koch-Weser, J. (1975) Ann. Intern. Med., 83, 237.
92. Greenblatt, D.J., Allen, M.D. and Shader, R.I. (1977) Clin. Pharmacol. Ther., 21, 355.
93. Hasegawa, M. and Matsurbara, I. (1975) Chem. Pharm. Bull. (Tokyo), 22, 1826.
94. deSilva, J.A.F. and Strojny, N. (1971) J. Pharm. Sci., 60, 1303.
95. Kaplan, S.A., de Silva, J.A.F., Jack, M.L., Alexander, K., Strojny, N., Weinfeld, R.E., Puglici, C.V. and Weissman, L. (1973) J. Pharm. Sci., 62, 1932.
96. Mahon, W.H., Inaba, T. and Stone, R.M. (1977) Clin. Pharmacol. Ther., 22, 228.
97. Greenblatt, D.J., Shader, R.I. and Koch-Weser, J. (1975) Clin. Pharmacol. Ther., 17, 1.
98. Kales, A., Bixler, E.O., Scharf, M. and Kales, J.D. (1976) Clin. Pharmacol. Ther., 19, 576.
99. Haider, I. (1968) Brit. J. Psychiatry, 114, 337.
100. Morgan, H., Scott, D.F. and Joyce, C.R.B. (1970) Brit. J. Psyciatry, 117, 649.
101. Linnoila, M. (1973) Ann. Med. Exp. Biol. Fenn., 51, 118.
102. Evans, J.G. and Jarvis, E.H. (1972) Brit. Med. J., 4, 487.
103. Castleden, C.M., George, C.F., Marcer, D. and Hallet, C. (1977) Brit. Med. J., 1, 10.
104. Linnoila, M. and Viukari, M. (1976) Brit. J. Psychiatry, 128, 566.
105. Kangas, L., Kanto, J., Siirtola, T. and Pekkarinen, A. (1977) Acta Pharmacol. Toxicol., 41, 74.
106. Kangas, L. (1979) Acta Pharmacol. Toxicol., 45, 16.
107. Reider, J. and Wendt, G. (1973) in Benzodiazepines. Garattini, S., Mussini, E. and Randall, L.O., ed., Raven Press, N.Y., pp. 99-127.
108.a Beyer, K.H. and Sadee, W. (1969) Forsch (Drug Research), 19, 1929.
109.a Karim, A.K.M.B. and Evans, D.A.P. (1976) J. Med. Genetics, 13, 17.
108.b Blackwell, B. (1975) Dis. Nerv. Syst., 36(5), Section 2, 17.
109.b Deberdt, R. (1978) Acta Psychiatr. Scand. Suppl., 274, 56.
110. Chesrow, E.J., Kaplitz, S.W., Vetra, H., Breme, J.T. and Marquardt, G.H. (1965) Clin. Med., 72, 1001.
111. Shull, H.J., Jr., Wilkinson, G.R., Johnson, R., Schenker, S. (1976). Ann. Int. Med., 84, 240.
112. Merlis, S. and Koepke, H.H. (1975) Dis. Nerv. Syst., 36(5), Section 2, 27.
113. Wilkinson, G.R. (1978) Acta Psychiate. Scand. Suppl., 274, 56.
114. Sisenwine, C.F., Tio, C.O., Sharader, S.R. and Ruelius, H.W. (1972) Arzneim-Forsch., 22, 682.
115. Conner, J.T., Parson, N., Katz, R.L., Wapner, S. and Bellville, J.W. (1976) Clin. Pharmacol. Ther., 19, 24.
116. Schillings, R.T., Shrader, S.R. and Ruelius, H.W. (1971) Arzneim-Forsch., 21, 1059.
117. Greenblatt, D.J., Shader, R.I., Franke, K., MacLaughlin, D.S., Harmatz, J.S., Allen, M.D.- Werner, A. and Woo, E. (1979) J. Pharm. Sci., 68, 57.
118. Greenblatt, D.J., Schillings, R.T., Kyriakopoulos, A.A., Shader, R.I., Sisenwine, S.F., Knowles, J.A. and Ruelius, H.W. (1976) Clin. Pharmacol. Ther., 20, 329.
119. Greenblatt, D.J., Joyce, T.H., Comer, W.H., Knowles, J.A., Shader, R.I., Kyriakopoulos, A.A., MacLaughlin, D.S. and Ruelius, H.W. (1977) Clin. Pharmacol. Ther., 21, 222.
120. Muller, W. and Wollert, U. (1973) Naunyn-Schmiedeberg's Arch. Pharmacol., 278, 301.
121. Rosenbaum, A.H., Maruta, T. and Richardson, E. (1979) Mayo Clinic Proc., 54, 401.

122. Small, J.G., Kellams, J.J., Milstein, V. and Moore, J. (1975) Amer. J. Psychiat., 132, 1315.
123. Amdisen, A. (1975) Danish Med. Bull., 22, 277.
124. Lehmann, K. and Merten, K. (1974) Int. J. Clin. Pharmacol., 10, 292.
125. Mason, R.W., McQueen, E.G., Keary, P.J. and James, N. McL. (1978) Clin. Pharmacokin., 3, 241.
126. Himmelhoch, J.M., Forrest, J., Neal, J.S. and Dedry, T.T. (1977) Amer. J. Psych., 34, 149.
127. Braestrup, C., Nielsen, M., Squires, R.F. and Laurberg, S. (1978) Acta Psychiatr. Scand. Suppl., 274, 27.
128. Mohler, H. and Okada, T. (1977) Life Sci., 20, 2102.
129. Mohler, H. and Okada, T. (1977) Science, 193, 849.
130. Squires, R.F. and Braestrup, C. (1977) Nature (London), 266, 732.
131. Regan, J., Roeske, W. and Yamamura, H. (1979) Pharmacologist 21, 149.
132. Mohler and Okada, 1978, in press.
133. Reisine, T.D., Wastek, G.J., Seth, R.C., Bird, E.D. and Yamaura, H.I. (1979) Brain Res., 165, 183.
134. Bender, A.D. (1964) J. Amer. Geriat. Sco., 12, 114.
135. Dwyer, B.E. and Wasterlain, C.G. (Oct. 5-7, 1978) Presented at the Eighth Annual National Meeting of the American Aging Association, San Francisco, CA.
136. Pearl, R. (1905) Biometrika, 4, 13.
137. Boyd, R. (1909) in Quain's Antomy, Shafer, A., Symington, J. and Bryce, T.H., ed., London, p. 342.
138. Minckler, T.M. and Boyd, E. (1968) in Pathology of the Nervous System, Vol. 1, Minkler, J., ed., New York, pp. 120-131.
139. Brizzee, K.R. (1975) in Neurobiology of Aging, Ordy, J.M. and Brizzee, E.M., ed., Plenum, New York, pp. 401-423.
140. Hall, T.C., Miller, A.K.H., Corsellis, J.A.N. (1975) Neuropathol. Appl. Neurobiol., 1, 267.
141. Andrew, W. (1971) The Anatomy of Aging in Man and Animals, Grune and Stratton, New York.
142. Ordy, J.M. and Kaack, B. (1975) in Neurobiology of Aging, Ordy, J.M. and Brizzee, R.R., ed., Plenum, New York, pp. 253-285.
143. Berlin, M. and Wallace, R.B. (1976) Exp. Aging Res., 2, 125.
144. Costa, E. and Guidotti, A. (1979) Ann. Rev. Pharmacol. Toxicol., 19, 531.
145. Bertilsson, L. (1978) Acta Psychiatr. Scand. Suppl., 274, 19.
146. Biggio, G., Brodie, B.B., Costra, E. and Guidotti, A. (1977) Proc. Natl. Acad. Sci. (USA), 74, 3592.
147. Kliner, L.M., Chi, Y.M., Friedberg, S.L., Rall, T.W. and Sutherland, E.W. (1962) J. Biol. Chem., 237, 1239.
148. Berndt, S. and Schwabe, U. (1973) Brain Res., 63, 303.
149. Schultz, J. (1979) Pharmacology, 18, 57.
150. Rutherford, D.M., Okoko, A., Tyrer, P.J. (1978) Brit. J. Clin. Pharmacol., 6, 69.
151. Greenblatt, D.J., Allen, M.D., Locniskar, A. and Shader, R.I. (1979) Clin. Pharmacol. Ther., 25, 227.

II
Evaluation and Management

THE PSYCHIATRIC EVALUATION OF THE GERIATRIC PATIENT

BESSEL A. VAN DER KOLK, M.D.
Staff Psychiatrist, Court Street V. A. Outpatient Clinic, Boston, MA
Assistant Clinical Professor of Psychiatry, Tufts University School of
Medicine

The elderly are a group with a disproportionate share of medical, emotional
and socioeconomic problems. About sixty percent of elderly people in the community suffer from at least mild emotional difficulties, and somewhere between
fifteen and twenty percent of the elderly population of the United States suffer
from moderate to severe psychopathology.[1,2,3] Approximately 125,000 elderly
patients reside in various mental hospitals to which the majority were first
admitted after age 65, while about 700,000 are residents in nursing homes.[4]
Butler[5] estimates that over one million elderly patients are institutionalized
at any particular time, while at least two million elderly people in the community suffer from chronic physical or mental problems. Unfortunately, with
the current trend to "deinstitutionalize" mental patients, geriatric patients
with psychiatric illnesses often are transferred from institutions with some
rehabilitation and treatment programs to nursing homes which serve a purely
custodial function. It is estimated that about eighty percent of nursing home
residents have moderate to severe psychiatric problems.[6]

Yet, the vast majority of people over 65, approximately 95%, continue to
live in the community where they display as much variability among themselves
as people in any other age group. Generally, the elderly continue to function
well within the framework of their previous personality makeup until one important traumatic event, or a series of smaller ones, disrupt their previous
adaptation.

The elderly are often exposed to multiple traumatic events which may occur
in brief succession: death of a spouse and contemporaries, decline in physical
health and prowess; loss of status, prestige and participation in society, and
a decline in standard of living which may condemn them to poverty with its
accompanying shame, stress, and lack of options. Not only do these disruptions
occur more frequently to the elderly, the elderly also tend to be less well
equipped to deal with them because of their depleted physiological, psychological and socioeconomic resources. Yet, it appears that the vast majority
of older people brace themselves for the vicissitudes which invariably accompany senescence. The work of Bernice Neugarten[7] suggests that most people tend

to be able to cope with anticipated events, almost no matter how traumatic, as long as they occur "on time." She suggests that "the psychology of the life cycle is the psychology not of crisis behavior, but the psychology of timing." The work of Zarit and Kahn[8] and Meyer[9] supports the view that old people tend to adapt to physical afflictions which occur "on time."

While many older people have an impressive capacity to deal with losses, it appears that an elderly person's health is most crucially related to his or her ability to bear up under stress.[10] It is estimated that 86% of people over 65 have one or more chronic illnesses, while 15% are unable to engage in a major activity.[11] While many elderly people spend a great deal of time and energy on what Butler calls "body monitoring," Ostfeld[12] found that only a relatively small percentage of older persons actually sought appropriate help for significant medical pathology.

Defenses

Psychological defenses against anxiety, rage and despair are called upon more than ever in coping with the losses of age and the preparation for death. In general, defense mechanisms remain stable, with some modifications, throughout life. However, there is a tendency among the elderly to rely on a somewhat more limited repertoire and somewhat more primitive psychological defenses[13] than before. Denial is a commonly used defense, particularly in old people with some degree of organic impairment. Denial, though useful in ignoring the unpleasant realities which the older person faces, can be a harmful mechanism of defense if it causes people not to seek medical, social, financial or psychiatric help for remediable conditions.

The use of the defense mechanism of projection also may increase with age, and is expressed in suspiciousness, feistiness, or paranoia. While the use of projection will markedly decrease a person's access to his environment, at least one study rated grouchiness and combativeness as a survival asset.[14]

While the obsessive compulsive defenses of isolation, reaction formation and displacement tend to be maladaptive earlier on, in the elderly they often provide structure and meaning to socially impoverished lives.[15] The use of these defenses also intensifies with age. People with schizoid or markedly introspective characters often adapt well to aging as they have already grown accustomed to leading independent lives with relatively little social interaction. Obsessive compulsive and schizoid people often do well as long as they can fend for themselves, but they are liable to get into conflicts with their environment, or to withdraw when forced in a more dependent position because of physical infirmities. People with passive dependent personalities tend to get into hostile dependent relationships with their environments when left to fend for themselves in old age, but they tend to make excellent adjustments when placed in institutions, where such behavior is usually encouraged and, in fact, counted on.

People with hysterical personalities or narcissistic characters who have been dependent on constant reassurance, praise or admiration, and who have managed to be the center of attention, the "life of the party," during their younger years, tend to have particularly severe reactions to accepting their aging selves and their new, diminished role in society. These people often become severely depressed and may present serious suicidal risks.[16,17,18]

In general, little personality change occurs as most people grow older until either major environmental changes occur, often an indirect result of physical disability or loss of social support, or until a person develops some degree of dementia. Most people who were relatively free of intrapsychic or interpersonal conflicts, who had ease in relating to their environment, and who had a sense of usefulness throughout their lives, will cope well even with physical illness, or mild degrees of cognitive impairment. Such people tend to deal with the realities of aging with positive action, and gain a sense of control over their lives by the use of insight and understanding of their condition and their surroundings. People with poorly resolved intrapsychic or interpersonal conflicts tend to rely on more primitive defenses and may undergo marked regression in the face of physical illness, uprooting from a previously familiar environment, or early cognitive deficits.

THE PSYCHIATRIC EVALUATION

Most elderly people are eager to talk about themselves in the context of a supportive environment. As a group, the elderly perform slower than younger people; pressure or uncertainty about the purpose of an interview are likely to bring out more confusion, anxiety, hostility, paranoia or shame than is necessary for an examiner to observe during a first interview. Since older people may be confused and disoriented in unfamiliar surroundings, it is important to clarify the nature and purpose of the evaluation, and to reassure the patient that the examiner is not there to declare the patient "crazy."

The psychiatric evaluation of older people does not differ in major ways from that of younger ones except that issues of physical health and capabilities, social support and economic well-being, accumulated life experience, attitude toward death, and issues of cognition play a generally more prominent role. It

may be more productive to have several brief interviews rather than one protracted one.

Influence of Physical Status

The physical status of the patient must always be carefully assessed. The
first encounter with the patient may reveal the physical signs of various illnesses with psychiatric concomitants. Parkinsonism is characterized by a mask-
like facies, and propulsive gait, with short, shuffling steps. Organicity may
reveal itself by physical incoordination as well as mental incoherence and ir-
relevance, and the appearance of premature aging and debilitation may point to
an underlying organic disease.

The initial evaluation of the elderly patient should include a physical examination, including chest x-rays, and laboratory studies for electrolytes,
thyroid, hepatic and renal function and serological tests for syphilis. As
specific diagnoses are entertained further laboratory studies may be indicated,
particularly in patients with symptoms of organic brain syndromes. Specifically, these include studies for Vitamin B_{12} deficiency, subdural hematoma, low
pressure hydrocephalus, and space occupying lesions in the brain. In addition,
sensory deficits should be carefully assessed. Deafness, in particular, may be
contributing to paranoid states, social isolation, and depression.

The Formal Mental Status Examination

A brief mental status examination and an assessment of social and psychological support systems should be routinely done as part of the medical evaluation of all elderly patients; it is as much an assessment of a patient's
neurological as his psychiatric condition.

A rough estimate of a patient's level of cognitive function can be obtained
by checking for orientation to time, place and person and testing for recent
memory. The latter is obtained by asking the patient to recall the names of
three objects, and the date, month, and year of the examination. More remote
memory can be checked by asking for the patient's home address and telephone
number, the names of his siblings and their children, or a patient's mother's
maiden name. If a somewhat more detailed testing of cognition is indicated,
left cerebral hemisphere function can be tested with serial sevens, and with
tests for digit span, backwards and forwards, while right hemisphere function
can be ascertained by asking the patient to draw a Greek cross, or to copy
various designs from the Bender-Gestalt test.

Psychological tests, particularly the WAIS, the Bender-Gestalt and the Halstead-Reitan, are very sensitive to organicity and may be helpful in both diagnosis and accurate measurement of the progress of cognitive deficits.

Whenever possible, an attempt should be made to establish a precipitant for the patient's contact with the evaluator. With the help of the patient's information, but if necessary by contacting family or friends, an evaluation should also be made of the patient's intelligence, prior level of functioning, and adaptive capabilities to role requirements.

Use of Family Informants

Contact with family or friends can be very illuminating about issues on which the patient lacks perspective, or which he needs to deny, or of which he may be ashamed. The patient may respond to pressures or conflicts within the family, or he may act out a role which the family has unconsciously assigned to him. It is not unusual that the patient is the victim of sibling rivalry in his children who either compete for the patient's favors, or who push the patient away onto other siblings who they feel have been favored more by the patient while growing up. Sometimes one may undercover a strong death wish on the part of children or other relatives of suicidal elderly patients, which may be the result of many years of unresolved family conflict. Family therapy with the relatives may help resolve some of these issues and relieve the unconscious pressures on the patient.

Assessment of Affect

The patient's feelings about his current life status should be examined, including attitudes toward activity, social contacts, living circumstances and economic issues. Vegetative signs of depression: loss of appetite, loss of libido, sleep disturbances, particularly early morning awakening, dry mouth and constipation should be specifically investigated. If the patient is found to be depressed, it is important to elicit a history of prior depressive episodes and their resolution, and to make an attempt to differentiate between chronic characterological depressions, unipolar depressions, or even bipolar manic depressive illness. It is useful to learn whether there is a depressive family history, and what treatment may have been successful.

Life Review

The life review provides the examiner with an assessment of the patient's object relations, his modes of adaptation to stress, the nature of possible identification figures, and his sense of values and accomplishments. In addition, it provides the patient with an often much needed opportunity to see his life in renewed perspective and to reminisce about past accomplishments and relationships.

TABLE 1

MEDICATIONS WHICH MAY CAUSE SYMPTOMS OF ORGANIC BRAIN SYNDROME

Anticholinergic agents--tricyclic antidepressants
                        antiparkinsonian medications
                        over the counter sleeping medication
                        antispasmodics
Analgesics--narcotics
            propoxyphene
            salicilate intoxication
Antimetabolites
Corticosteroids
Digitalis compounds
Psychic stimulants--amphetamines
                    methylphenidate
Psychotropic drugs--antipsychotic agents
                    antianxiety agents
Antiparkinsonian agents--L-Dopa
                         carbidopa
Methyldopa
Methysergide

TABLE 2

MEDICATIONS WHICH MAY CAUSE OR AGGRAVATE DEPRESSION

Antihypertensive agents--reserpine
                         methyldopa
                         propanolol
                         guanethidine
                         hydralazine
Antiparkinsonian agents--L-Dopa
                         bromocriptine
                         carbidopa
Corticosteroids
Antimetabolites
Digitalis compounds
Antipsychotics
Antidepressants
Antianxiety agents

Medication Evaluation

The patient, and if necessary people in his environment, should be questioned in a detailed fashion about all prescription drugs, over the counter medications, and recreational chemicals (mainly alcohol) which he may be taking. Numerous medications may cause or aggravate symptoms of organic brain syndrome (see Table 1), or precipitate or aggravate depression (see Table 2).

Treatment Plan

At the end of the psychiatric examination, a decision needs to be made whether a patient has the psychological capacity to maintain an independent role in the community. If not, provisions need to be made, if possible in consultation with the patient and the family, for placement of the patient in a more supportive environment. Clarity and preparation are crucial if this decision is taken. Prevarication and ambiguity in the environment may greatly increase disorientation and confusion in brain damaged patients, and may easily lead to the Goldstein catastrophic reaction in which the patient is flooded with anxiety and panic.

Usually, less drastic steps are necessary, and the treatment plan may vary from the provision of warm meals, or the linking up with a senior citizen's club, to psychotherapy or pharmacotherapy.

PSYCHOPATHOLOGY

Affective Disorders

More than half of all elderly patients seen in mental health centers suffer from depressions, mainly involutional melancholias or neurotic depressions. These disorders are characterized by feelings of helplessness, hopelessness and worthlessness, apathy, sadness, loneliness, boredom, and lack of sexual interest in the patient. The mental symptoms of depression frequently are accompanied by the so-called vegetative signs: insomnia, particularly early morning awakening, loss of appetite, dryness of the mouth and constipation.

The elderly tend to be particularly vulnerable to depression, not only because of psychological and socioeconomic reasons, but probably also because of biological factors, such as an increase in brain monamine oxidase[19] and a decrease in cerebral norepinephrine and dopamine.[20] Many people who have not experienced depressions during their adult life have severely depressed episodes during senescence. Busse[21] has pointed out a close relationship between decline in physical health and depression. For many older people the loss of physical health is harder to bear than the loss of love objects or prestige;

not only does physical decline hurt an old person's self respect, it also may easily lead to social isolation.

Butler[5] points out that guilt, as well as decreased self-regard is an important causative factor in depression in the elderly. He emphasizes that older people are still capable of actions which provoke guilt, and that in reviewing their lives elderly people are sometimes tormented by remorse over past actions. Other writers find older depressed patients less preoccupied with guilt feelings than younger ones.

Involutional melancholia is a psychotic depressive reaction which occurs first between the ages of 45 and 65, generally somewhat earlier in women than in men, in people who generally have had adequate previous life adjustments. The depressive affect is profound, and is usually accompanied by delusions of guilt or somatic delusions, and sometimes by hallucinations. This form of depression usually responds very well to tricyclic antidepressants or electroshock treatment.

Pathological Grief Reactions

Mourning the loss of a loved one usually requires from 3 to 12 months prior to resolution.[22] It is not uncommon for elderly people to cope with the loss of a loved one, not by mourning, but by idealization, which entails an "enshrinement"[5] of the loved one at the exclusion of new attachments. The conflict underlying this idealization is related to unconscious hostility toward the loved one, survival guilt, and fear of being blamed for infidelity if investment in new relationships occurs.

Another form of pathological mourning occurs when no conscious mourning of the lost love occurs, but the survivor defends himself against the conscious experience of grief by means of identification with the somatic symptoms of the loved one.

Mourning may be less complete in older people because there is less hope for renewal of attachments.

Memory Impairment and Depression

Memory impairment is a frequent complaint with which elderly patients present themselves to the physician. Usually, little correlation is found between the degree of cognitive impairment, psychological testing and the seriousness of the subjective experience of the patient. Patients whose psychological test results reveal much less memory impairment than suggested by the initial complaint tend to be depressed.[23] It appears that memory impairment is exaggerated by people with normal brain function who are depressed, while people with true organic deficits tend to minimize their difficulties.[24]

Mild, reversible memory changes are frequently found in depressed patients[25], while more severe memory loss is found in pseudodementia,[26] where patients appear confused and disoriented in addition to their memory loss. Unlike in true dementia, the onset is quite abrupt, usually after a precipitating loss. Rather than confabulation, patients with this syndrome display negativism and hostility upon questioning. Pseudodementia tends to occur in people with limited intelligence.

The tricyclic antidepressants have potent anticholinergic side effects which may themselves cause confusion and memory impairment, particularly in elderly patients.[27] In one study with depressed elderly patients with mild to moderate memory impairment, Hydergine 1 mg. t.i.d. was found to have almost as potent antidepressant activity as imipramine, without its concomitant anticholinergic side effects.[28]

Depressive Equivalents

Depressive equivalents usually occur in previously successful people who rather late in life develop sudden severe pain, usually in the back, neck or head. These patients usually only feel depressed about the occurrence of the pain which they experience as a personal failure. Only after no organic basis for the pain is found and a precipitating loss is uncovered does it become clear that the patient is experiencing a depression.[29]

Somatization and Hypochondriasis

With the high incidence of physical problems in the elderly, it is not surprising that preoccupation with bodily functions plays a more prominent role than in younger people. In at least one study, 30% of elderly patients were found to have high bodily concern, and of these, one-third was found to have neurotically based somatic concerns. Somatization is a common psychological defense which older people use to deal with problems about dependence and responsibility. Busse[11] has pointed out that the assumption of the sick role absolves the patient of the socially expected need for independence, financial success, and social prestige. While people with emotional problems tend to be held responsible for the state they find themselves in, physically ill people generally are viewed by themselves and others as victims of circumstances over which they have no control, but which they heroically struggle to overcome. Hypochondriasis tends to occur in older people, especially women, who experience real or imagined neglect from their families. As Pfeiffer[4] points out: "the interactional world has become unrewarding and hostile for the hypochondriacal patient, and...she has turned instead towards...her own body as an interesting theater for observation."

The hypochondriacal older person experiences his physical ills as a valuable means of communicating with the outside world, and as a link with family members and health care providers. Dismissing a patient's complaint with reassurance is experienced as a rejection and is followed by either an escalation of physical complaints, or, more seldom, anger or withdrawal. Treatment is slow and painstaking, but may meet with some success if more mutually rewarding relationships can be substituted for the hostile dependent ones which usually accompany hypochondriasis.

Psychophysiological Disorders

In contrast to hypochondriasis, psychophysiological disorders are accompanied by definite organic changes which are a real threat to the patient. Unlike conversion reactions, these physical symptoms provide no relief from anxiety, and there is a physiological, rather than a symbolic origin of the symptoms.[30] Common psychophysiological reactions among the elderly are pruritus ani and vulvae, irritable colon, psychogenic components of rheumatism and hyperventilation syndromes. Psychotherapy tends to be helpful in alleviating the severity of the symptoms.

Adjustment Reactions

Even mildly organically impaired people are prone to react to stressful situations with unmodified anxiety. Fear, confusion, agitation and pressure of speech may be the presenting difficulty together with such somatic symptoms as shortness of breath, rapid pulse rate, tremulousness, and disturbed sleep.

These patients experience a great need to ventilate and repeatedly recount the traumatic event. The benzodiazepines may be useful in alleviating the distress, but caution should be exercised to keep the dosages small, and to restrict their use to the duration of the episode so as to prevent drug habituation, and the psychological and physiological side effects to which the elderly are prone.

Jarvik and Russell[31] point out that in addition to gross anxiety, paranoia, or withdrawal in reaction to emergancy situations, the elderly may employ a passive stance, called "freeze," in the face of stressful events over which they have no control. The passive stance of "freeze" allows the elderly greater adaptive flexibility than the "fight" or "flight" reactions more commonly employed in younger people.

Paranoid Reactions

Solitary living, social isolation, sensory deficits, particularly deafness, and a general inability to interpret the meaning of new information frequently give rise to various degrees of paranoia in the elderly. Projection, the defense mechanism underlying paranoia, is very common in the elderly, and in and of itself is not a measure of severe psychopathology in this age group. The severity of the paranoia ranges from mild paranoid reactions, particularly at night, to full-blown paranoid psychoses, often in people with concomitant organic brain syndrome. Ten percent of geriatric psychiatric admissions have paranoia as their principal precipitant.[32]

Since helplessness and disorientation are the underlying causes of paranoid reactions, environmental manipulations such as increased aid in coping with the demands of daily living, orienting stimuli, such as night lights, an increase in consistency in the environment, or the alleviation of sensory deficits, for example by giving a deaf person a hearing aid, may go a long way to decreasing the paranoia. Psychotherapy can be helpful. Antipsychotic medications may help a great deal in modifying the paranoia, but as drugs themselves are frequently subject to suspicion, drug compliance is very low, except when either administered in a protective setting or by a trusted person.

Schizophrenia in Later Life

Numerous deinstitutionalized older schizophrenics now inhabit our nursing homes and hospitals for the aged. They frequently are more the end products of long institutional regression than of their illness per se. Older schizophrenics rarely are grossly psychotic and many do quite well without any antipsychotic medications.

Recent work[33,34] has disproved the notion that schizophrenia always is a chronically deteriorating process leading to cognitive impairment and affective impoverishment. Many older schizophrenics, unless victims of chronic institutionalization, tend to become more affectively engaged with their surroundings and display a greater ability to fend for themselves than at an earlier age.

Suicide in the Elderly

The elderly, about ten percent of the population, account for roughly twenty-five percent of suicides.[35] The rate of suicide increases steadily in

white males, to reach a peak incidence of 45 per 100,000 after age 80. Women
have a somewhat lower incidence which reaches its peak in late middle age at
13 per 100,000 after which it declines. The elderly black population has a
lower incidence of suicide than its white counterpart, but there has been a
substantial increase over the past two decades.

Elderly people generally give little warning prior to suicide and attempts
seldom fail.[36] Manipulation of the environment or a desire for revenge rarely
seem to be a motivating factor in elderly suicides. Isolation, alcoholism,
recent bereavement, physical illness, insomnia, induced helplessness and depression are frequent precipitating factors. Older people often give very
little indication of their suicidal intent. Increased withdrawal, an increase
in alcohol consumption or an uncharacteristic preoccupation with physical
symptoms sometimes are warning signs, particularly in single elderly men.

ORGANIC BRAIN SYNDROMES

Organic brain syndromes due to brain cell death or brain cell malfunction
contribute to almost fifty percent of the behavioral disturbances seen in
patients over 65 years of age.[37] Numerous pathological processes may underlie
the behavioral syndrome referred to as organic brain syndrome: Alzheimer's
Disease, Pick's Disease, cerebrovascular malfunction, low pressure hydrocephalus, space occupying lesions, Huntington's Chorea and various metabolic
and infectious processes.

Most people with organic brain syndromes come to the attention of physicians
because of behavior that is disturbing to relatives and friends, rather than
because of subjective distress. The clinical presentation of these various
pathological processes is uniform enough to make specific diagnoses on the
basis of behavioral observations or cognitive functioning alone impossible. The
degree of behavioral disturbance or cognitive impairment is no accurate indication of the degree of brain impairment since premorbid personality, motivation, cooperativeness and environmental factors impact heavily on the
behavioral expression of organic impairment.[38]

The basic behavioral manifestations of cerebral impairment are memory loss,
disorientation, confusion, loss of intellectual functions such as comprehension,
problem solving, learning and judgment, as well as emotional lability, and
restlessness or withdrawal and unresponsiveness.

Reversible versus Irreversible Syndromes

While the majority of older patients with organic brain syndrome suffer from
Alzheimer's Disease or Senile Dementia, and about twenty percent from cerebrovascular impairment, about twenty percent have a condition which is reversible,
or which at least can be arrested if diagnosed early. These correctible disorders include drug toxicity, normal pressure hydrocephalus, benign intracranial masses, mania, thyroid disease, pernicious anemia, epilepsy and hepatic
failure. Brain disease secondary to hypertension, alcohol and syphilis can at
least be palliated if diagnosed early.

The consistent finding that about fifteen to twenty percent of people who
present with the symptoms of an organic brain syndrome have reversible pathology[39,40,41] makes an attempt to establish the etiology of the organic brain
syndrome imperative.

Senile Dementia and Alzheimer's Disease

Senile dementia, a syndrome consisting of neuronal loss and the appearance
of new structural elements in the brain, is probably the same pathological
entity which, if it appears at a younger age, is called Alzheimer's Disease.
It is a slowly progressive dementia which has genetic components, though the
genetic data on senile dementia and on Alzheimer's disease are not in strict
agreement. One study claims that senile dementia is determined by a single
autosomal dominant gene carried by about 12% of the population. Its penetrance
appears to increase with age until it reaches 40% manifestation at age 90.[42]
Concordance for senile dementia occurs in 43% of monozygotic and 8% of dizy-
gotic twins.[44]

The average life expectancy for people admitted to the hospital with senile
dementia is 2 years. There is progressive deterioration with a slow break up
of speech into fragmented phrases, logorrhea and dysphasias. Most patients
show an utter disinterest in their surroundings, but about one-third display
behavior disturbances including aimless wandering, assaultiveness, or persistent screaming. The practice of prescribing unnecessary psychotropic
medications may contribute to the high incidence of falls and fractures in
this population.[45] Resulting subdural hematomas may easily be overlooked in
patients with preexisting dementia and confusion.

Arteriosclerotic Brain Disease

While on autopsy 20% of demented elderly patients are found to have pathological changes typical of both senile dementia and cerebrovascular disease,[11]

most people with arteriosclerotic brain disease present with a rather different
clinical picture than people with senile dementia.

Senile dementia affects two-and-one-half times more women than men,
while the prevalence of arteriosclerotic dementia is the opposite. Some
investigators believe that female hormones may play a protective role against
cerebrovascular disease.[11]

The underlying pathology consists of focal brain lesions due to vascular
occlusions and concomitant focal neurological signs are usually found. The
onset is most commonly abrupt and the course is fluctuating. This is due in
part to the fact that the edema which occurs around the infarcted area re-
solves over time, while small arteriolar occlusions continue to take their
toll on functioning brain tissue. Usually, other arteriosclerotic changes
can be found elsewhere in the body.

People with cerebrovascular lesions tend to have a better preservation of
their personalities than patients with senile dementia. They often maintain
a degree of insight and depression is quite common.

Since there is some hope for effective palliation or treatment of
cerebrovascular disease, as discussed elsewhere in this volume, an attempt
should be made to make an accurate differential diagnosis between senile
dementia and cerebral arteriosclerotic disease. Cerebral arteriography
and computerized axial tomography are two particularly useful diagnostic
tools.

ACKNOWLEDGMENTS

The author wishes to acknowledge the help of Dr. Martin Merovitz in the
preparation of this manuscript.

REFERENCES
1. Srole, L., Langner, T.S., Michael, S.T., Opler, M.K. and Rennie, T.A.C.
(1962) Mental Health in the Metropolis: The Midtown Manhattan Study.
McGraw-Hill, New York.
2. Lowenthal, M.F., Bisette, G.G., Buehler, J.A., Pierce, R.C., Robinson, B.C.
and Iner, M.L. (1967) Aging and Mental Disorder in San Francisco. Jossey-
Bass, San Francisco.
3. Kay, D.W.K., Beamish, P. and Roth, M. (1964) Br. J. Psychiat. 465, 146-158.
4. Pfeiffer, E. (1977) in Handbook of the Psychology of Aging, Birren, J.E.
and Schaie, K.W., ed., Van Nostrand Reinhold, New York, pp. 650-671.
5. Butler, R.N. and Lewis, M.I. (1977) Aging and Mental Health, The C. V.
Mosby Company, St. Louis, pp. 52-53.
6. Teeter, R.B., Garetz, F.K., Miller, W.R. and Heiland, W.F. (1976) Am. J.
Psychiat. 133, 1430-1434.
7. Neugarten, B.L. (1970) J. Geriat. Psychiat. 4, 71-100.
8. Zarit, S.H. and Kahn, R.L. (1975) J. Gerontol. 30, 67-72.

9. Meyer, G.G. (1974) in Psychological Basis of Medical Practice: An Introduction to human behavior, Bowden, C.L. and Burstein, A.G., eds., Williams and Williams, Baltimore, pp. 203-214.
10. Eisdorfer, C. and Wilkie, F. (1977) in Handbook of the Psychology of Aging, Birren, J.E. and Schaie, K.W., eds., Van Nostrand Reinhold, New York, pp. 251-270.
11. Busse, E.W. (1973) in Mental Illness in Later Life, Busse, E.W. and Pfeiffer, E., eds., American Psychiatric Association, Washington, D.C., pp. 89-106.
12. Ostfeld, A.M. (1968) in The Retirement Process, Carp, F.M., ed., U.S. Dept. HEW (US PHS Publ. No. 1778), Washington, D.C., pp. 83-96.
13. Vaillant, G.E. (1971) Arch Gen. Psychiat. 24, 107-118.
14. Lieberman, M.A. (1975) in Life Span Developmental Psychology: Normative Life Crises, Datan, N. and Ginsberg, L., eds., Academic Press, New York.
15. Perlin, S. and Butler, R.N. (1963) in Human Aging, Birren, J.E., Butler, R.N., Greenhouse, S.W., Sokoloff, L. and Yarrow, M.R., eds., U.S. Government Printing Office, Publication No. (HSM) 71-9051, Washington, D.C., pp. 159-217.
16. Blau, D. and Berezin, M.A. (1975) in Modern Perspectives in the Psychiatry of Old Age, Howells, John G., ed., Brunner, Mazel, New York, pp. 201-233.
17. Levin, S. (1965) Int. J. Psychoanal. 46, 200-205.
18. Zarsky, E.L. and Blau, D. (1970) J. Geriat. Psychiat. 3, 160-164.
19. Robinson, D.S. (1975) Federation Proceedings 34, 103-107.
20. Gottfries, G.G., Gottfries, I., Johnson, B., Olson, R., Persson, T., Roos, B.E. and Sjöström, R. (1971) Neuropharmacology 10, 665-672.
21. Busse, E.W. (1968) International Mental Health Research Newsletter 10, 13-16.
22. Lindemann, E. (1944) Amer. J. Psychiat. 101, 141-148.
23. Beck, A.T. (1967) Depression. Hoeber, New York.
24. Kahn, R.L., Zarit, S.H., Hilbert, N.M. and Niederche, G. (1975) Arch Gen. Psychiat. 32, 1569-1573.
25. Grinker, R.R., Miller, J. and Shabshin, M. (1961) The Phenomena of Depression. Paul B. Hoeber, Inc., New York.
26. Kiloh, L.G. (1961) Acta Psychiat. Scand. 37, 336-351.
27. van der Kolk, B.A., Shader, R.I. and Greenblatt, D.J. (1977) in Psychopharmacology, a Generation of Progress, Lipton, M.A., DiMascio, A. and Killam, K., eds., Raven Press, New York, pp. 1009-1016.
28. Shader, R.I., Harmatz, J. and van der Kolk, B.A. (1976) Unpublished manuscript.
29. Gallemore, J.L. and Wilson, W.P. (1969). Southern Med. J. 62, 551-555.
30. Maddox, G.L. (1964) J. Chronic Dis. 17, 449-460.
31. Jarvik, L.F. and Russell, D. (1979) J. of Gerontology 34, 197-200.
32. Post, F. (1966) Persistent Persecutory States of the Elderly. Pergamon, London.
33. Bridge, T.P., Cannon, H.E. and Wyatt, R.J. (1978) J. of Geront. 33, 835-839.
34. Bleuler, M. (1979) The Schizophrenic Disorders: Long Term Patient and Family Studies. Yale University Press, New Haven, Conn.
35. Resnick, H.L. and Cantor, J.M. (1970) J. Am. Gerat. Soc. 18, 152-158.
36. O'Neil, P., Robins, E. and Schmidt, E.H. (1956) AMA Arch. Neurol. Psychiat. 75, 275-284.
37. Kramer, M., Taube, C., and Redick, R. (1973) in The Psychology of Adult Development and Aging, Eisdorfer, C. and Lawton, M.P., eds., American Psychological Association, Washington, D.C.
38. Wang, H.S. (1973) in Mental Illness in Later Life, Busse, E.W. and Pfeiffer, E., eds., American Psychiatric Association, Washington, D.C., pp. 77-88.
39. Marsden, C.D. and Harrison, M.J.G. (1972) Br. Med. J. 2, 249-252.
40. Nott, P.N. and Fleminger, J.J. (1975) Acta Psychiatr. Scand. 51, 210-217.

41. Engel, G.L. and Romano, J. (1959) J. Chron. Diseases 9, 260-277.
42. Larson, T., Sjögren, T. and Jacobson, G. (1963) Acta Psychiat. Scand. 39 (Suppl. 167).
43. Pratt, R.T.C. (1970) in Alzheimer's Disease and Related Conditions, Walstenholme, G.E.W. and O'Connor, M., eds., Ciba, London, pp. 137-139.
44. Roth, M. (1955) J. Ment. Sci. 101, 281-285.
45. Rosin, A.J. (1977) Gerontology 23, 37-46.

Published 1979 by Elsevier North Holland, Inc.
Nandy, Ed. Geriatric Psychopharmacology

NEUROLOGICAL EVALUATION OF GERIATRIC PATIENTS WITH DEMENTIA AND RELATED

DISORDERS

MICHAEL J. MALONE, M.D.
Geriatric Research, Education and Clinical Center, Veterans Administration
Hospital, Bedford, Massachusetts and Boston University School of Medicine,
Boston, Massachusetts, USA.

There are myriad illnesses capable of causing protracted disability for the

aged person but none pose the spector of reason and identity loss which con-

fronts patients with dementia. Recent estimates indicate that there are

over 1.2 million individuals currently hospitalized in nursing homes and

other long-term care facilities. The greatest number of these patients are

hospitalized with such diagnoses as senility, dementia and stroke. In the

Medical Services of the Veterans Administration, over thirty thousand patients

are hospitalized with the diagnosis of senile dementia and this number is

expected to triple within the next two decades[1]. Senescent change may involve

a variety of clinical presentations. The most obvious is an alteration in

behavior.

This behavioral change can range from transient confusion and withdrawal

to gross disorientation and memory loss. In some cases, the cause is

primarily affective or functional. In others, organic changes ranging from

mild metabolic impairments to regional degeneration in the central nervous

system constitute the underlying etiology.

Presentation: The patient is most frequently seen in a physicians office

because of behavioral change. In most cases, early dementing change is

slow and overt manifestations are subtle. Even patients who are integral

parts of close families can frequently sink to gross levels of mental

incapacity before their condition is noted. Dementia refers to a loss of

mental faculties. This loss involves an inability to learn - to store and retrieve data, to affirm identities or dissimilarities, to generalize or abstract - and to plan effectively for future change. Probably, the earliest faculties to be affected limit an individual in his ability to form proper judgments in complex professional areas and this is reflected in early occupation problems - the sales manager whose record is declining, the loan officer whose risk assessments have become questionable. At this stage, neither formal testing nor clinical examination is likely to be revealing and the patient's perception of his disabilities may prompt a depressive reaction. In social circumstances, the patient's family or friends may be aware of personality changes reflected in recreational interests, blunting of affect and a lessened 'sense of humor.' Gradual changes in memory follow. The patients are unable to recall, first, the names of recent acquaintances then the identities of old friends, and finally confuse members of their own families.

In this context, the term confusion is defined as a situation or condition marked by a lack of order, system or arrangement[2]. If orderly though processes are in disarray, the patient will be unable to maintain his proper references in terms of space, time and ultimately in terms of his own person. This disorientation and confusion may appear in the end stage of a severe dementia, become superimposed on a mild dementia or appear as a transient reaction to exogenous (drugs) or endogenous (metabolic) toxins.

Evaluation: Documentation of the patient's illness is the first step in evaluation. It is critically important to decide whether or not the changes leading to presentation were gradual or sudden in onset. Frequently, a family member will date all events from some sudden change such as episode of trauma or singularly inappropriate behavior. Elderly persons, even while living at home, may have limited inter-relationships with active family members. Such social isolation can result in a failure to note advanced mental deterioration. In this context, information concerning the patient's occupation or hobbies may be objective and invaluable. Specific information should be sought in order to assess the rate of progress and details concerning episodes of memory loss, spacial disorientation and questionable judgments assist this assessment. The status of mood changes can be sought from the patient and other family members and the examiner should be most attentive to mood changes which are at variance with the patient's past personality.

In terms of past medical history, the examiner usually documents past neurological, caridorespiratory, gastrointestinal and other visceral organ ailments. In addition to careful listing of prescribed medications, it is essential to remember that elderly individuals are prone to multiple drug usage and many such drugs - laxatives, antacids, analgesics - can be purchased without prescription and used in gross excess.

In system review, an effort should be made to exclude symptoms of cerebro-vascular insufficiency - transient impairments of speech, vision or consicous-ness, episodes of vertigo or syncope. A detailed review of exercise tolerance, breathing difficulties, chest pain or palpitation should be obtained from the patient or his family. The patient's appetite and food intake should be recorded and particular attention given to dietary idiosyncracies and habitual use of antacids or laxative preparations. It is noteworthy that many depressed elderly patients will offer multiple somatic complaints with a particular focus on the gastrointestinal system (constipation, obstipation). Although tic douloureux is a rare entity, complaints of atypical facial pain are common in depressed individuals.

A general physical examination should be made and the examiner should test carefully for evidence of peripheral vascular problems, emphysema and border-line states of congestive heart failure.

Neurological Examination: Examination of the nervous system in aged or
demented patients (and these terms are not synonymous) is difficult and
frequently time-consuming. First, is the clinical assessment of mental states.
It is important to determine the specific degree of alertness demonstrated
by the patient and to distinguish a normal alert state from lethargy and
stupor or obtundation. The orientation of the patient to person, place,
time and circumstances must be noted. Memory should be tested in terms of
immediate recall, recent and remote memory functions. Finally, the ability
of the patient to identify similarities versus dissimilarities and to form
abstract concept should be documented by standard bedside testing methods[3].
Examination of the cranial nerves is usually carried out next followed by
evaluation of the motor system. This examination proceeds from inspection
for abnormal movements or atrophy to assessment of passive terms, strength
and elicitation of deep muscle reflexes. Pathological reflexes, indicative
of cortico-spinal tract dysfunction should be tested and coordination functions
determined on an equilibratory/non-equilibratory basis. Sensory modalities –
primary pain, temperature, touch and vibration – position sense-estimations
are made. Only then should the examiner review the patient's ability to
associate primary modalities to form judgments of form, shape and identity,
and to communicate his concepts in meaningful fashion. Specific changes in
the neurological examination of elderly subjects have been reviewed by
Paulson[4].

Testing:

   1. If the patient shows evidence of diffuse memory loss, spatial confusion
and limited ability to generalize or abstract a clinical testing, further
evaluation by psychometric testing may be useful either to define the problem
in more precise terms or to serve as a standard for future reference.
Useful standard testing devices include the Wechsler Adult Intelligence

Scale (WAIS), the Bender-Gestalt and Goldstein-Scheerer Test of Abstract and Concrete Thinking, the Wechsler Memory Scale[5]. On these tests, all scores are lowered in moderate to severe dementia - usually with greater impairment of verbal versus performance scores on the WAIS.

2. The Electroencephalogram: The clinical EEG is usually included in clinical evaluation of patients who present with behavioral change. The test is non-invasive and has maximum value in exclusion of focal brain disease. A generalized slowing in overall EEG frequencies with lesser alpha activity and increasing theta slowing bilaterally in frontal and temporo-occipital regions is generally seen in elderly individuals[6a&b]. In dementing disorders, the changes in EEG are dependent on the stage of the degenerative process, but the changes do not correlat well with clinical features. Normal EEG records have been reported in the presence of documented mental change. Generally, in advanced dementia there is an accentuation of features found in normal elderly populations. The records are characterized by an absence of alpha activity, generalized low voltage slowing into the theta and even delta frequencies and no focal features[7].

3. Radiological Studies: X-ray studies of the skull in other than trauma and states of abnormal calcification have little relevance in the study of behavioral change. Contrast studies - cerebral angiography and pneumo-encephalography - are invasive and have a significant morbidity in elderly patients. The introduction of Computerized Axial Tomography (CAT), based on density analyses by Oldendorf[8] and developed by Hounsfield[9], has raised the promise of an invaluable non-invasive diagnostic tool. The clinical value of the CAT scan in focal neurological disorders (infarction, hemorrhage, abscess, tumor) has had excellent clinicopathological documentation[10]. However the changes observed in 'normal' aged human brains (diminished brain weight) atrophy of gyri, widening of sulci and ventricular dilation seem to

show quantitative rather than qualitative differences when compared with the changes observed in senile dementia[11],[12]. Thus, the radiologic finding of brain atrophy may not correlate well with the clinical presentation. This problem is more apt to arise in differential considerations between demented and depressed patients.

4. Laboratory Studies: The general purpose of clinical laboratory studies is to confirm or deny the presence of metabolic derrangements. In the elderly patient, the choice of specific tests is dictated by the general medical evaluation results. Dehydration and inadequate nutrition may be reflected in the admission hemogram, electrolyte determinations and in plasma protein levels. Hypothyroidism can be screened by measurement of serum, T_3-T_4 levels and under the circumstances of anemia, clinical poly-neuropathy and dementia, serum folate and B_{12} levels are useful. It is important to note that many aberrations from standard laboratory values may be encountered in an aged population. These variations can arise from concomitant drug intake and from age-related variations in normative values. This subject has been reviewed recently by Hodkinson[13].

Differential Diagnosis

Faced with the presentation of an altered behavioral state, the examiner must distinguish initially between the following possibilities: First, an acute confusional state or delirium in an otherwise intact individual. Secondly, a confusional state aggravating a mild or moderate dementia. Third, a dementia without significant functional overlay and finally, a functional depression with little, if any, intellectual deterioration.

The individual who is essentially in an acute confused state lacks ability to concentrate and focus attention. The stream of language and though is rambling and tengential. The patient is distracted and distractable. Inattention leads to disorientation and fluctuating memory loss. The specific memory loss, however, associated with Korsakoff's Syndrome is not present and the consistent global loss of abstraction and all memory functions encountered in dementia is not present in patients suffering from acute confusional states. Moreover, the level of conciousness is usually altered and dependent on the etiology of the confusional state, the patient may be agitated, lethargic or stuporous. In states of acute intoxication the patient may misperceive reality and hallucinations - characteristically visual - may appear. Differential considerations include:

A. Toxic states

    1. Endogenous or metabolic

        a. hypercapnia, hypoxia (COPD, cardiac decompensation)

        b. hypoglycemia (insulin related)

        c. disorders of electrolyte balance and screen pH

        d. visceral organ failure: uremia, hepatic encephalopathy, endocrinopathies

        e. acute/subacute vitamin deficiency states (thiamine)

    2. Exogenous

        a. Ethanol intoxications

        b. Drug or iatrogenic intoxication - in this category - the examiner should be aware of the propensity for self medication (soporifics, laxatives) on the part of older patients.

B. Infectious processes

    1. Septicemia-meningitis, encephalitis

C. Trauma

    1. Status post head trauma, ictal, post-ictal states and in the acute phase of cerebral vascular accidents.

After exclusion of these conditions and with historical evidence for progressive mental deterioration, the mental status examination, followed by psychometric testing should document dementia. This is a symptom, the cause of which must be determined by the clinician. For the purpose of nosology, differential considerations can be organized as follows:

a. Dementia occurring secondary to focal or multifocal lesions. In this group, dementia appears in association with evidence of other neurological deficits - motor, sensory or disturbances of localizable cortical functions.

(1) Vascular

(a) Gross disturbance of brain function by massive infarction or hemorrhage will be accompanied early by alterations in the level of conciousness. In chronic cases, dementia may be a concomitant finding. Relatively minor infarcts particularly when the right parietal lobe or bilateral involvement of inferomedial portions of the occipital lobe (grenzgebieten) can result in dementia. The neurological examination will document focal motor or sensory deficits in these patients.

(b) Multiple small infarctions (multi-infarct dementia) occurring in the course, e.g., of systemic hypertension can produce a clinical picture very similar to a primary dementia. However, if a detailed history can be obtained, the examiner may be able to document the episodic nature of onset and CAT scan procedures can be useful.

(2) Metabolic

(a) Certain deficiency states (B_{12} folate) will produce a state of dementia associated with other neurological abnormalities and these are diagnosed by specific clinical chemistry studies.

(3) Neoplastic

(a) Gliomas, maningiomas. These mass lesions are associated with dementia (which may be a relatively early finding when primary tumors begin in fronto-temporal areas) as well as focal neurological

signs and evidence of increased intracranial pressure.

(4) Infectious processes

(a) Chronic granulomatous infections such as tuberculosis

and fungal meningitis. These tend to be basal in origin and impede the

absorption of cerebrospinal fluid. Other basal meningites - secondary to

sarcoidosis, carcinomatous involvement of the meninges - enter as diagnostic

considerations. Diagnosis may be difficult and dependent on cerebrospinal

fluid finding, the results of radio-isotope scans and in some cases,

surgical biopsy results.

(5) Normal Pressure Hydrocephalus

(a) This disorder occurs as a progressive dementia

usually associated with significant motor or higher cortical function

(apraxias) impairment. In some cases, a past history of meningitis or sub-

arachnoid hemorrhage may be obtained. Diagnosis is based on demonstration

of impaired cerebrospinal fluid flow and absorption on radioisotope scans

(cisternography). Since this is a potentially treatable condition, every

effort should be made to exclude such a possibility in patients with progres-

sive dementia.

(6) Pseudo-dementia is a term used in reference to a group

of patients whose clinical presentations resemble dementia in terms of

social withdrawal and psychomotor delay. Depressive reactions are the most

common problems in this group. Clinical distinction from dementia is

suggested by the following features:

(a) A past history of psychiatric illness

(b) An ability to date symptom onset with considerable

precision by the patient and/or his family - usually in relationship

to social or personal loss

(c) A pronounced tendency on the patients' part to
emphasize such symptoms as memory loss or disorientation.

(d) On mental status testing, these patients demonstrate
memory loss which is frequently selective rather than global and varies
in performance on repetetive testing. A useful rating scale for differentiation of pseudo-dementia from dementia has been developed by Wells[14].

(7) Dementia of the senile or pre-senile (Alzheimer) type,
as a degenerative disorder of unknown etiology, is the most commonly encountered neurological disorder in an older population[15, 16, 17, 18]. The
clinical presentation and findings on examination have been reviewed extensively
by Seltzer and co-workers[19, 20]. In general, historical review usually notes
that an exact date of symptom onset is very difficult to ascertain. In
fact, many families are unaware of change until symptoms are far advanced
(possibly a comment on the level of intra-familial communication).
Progression of symptoms is usually slow unless changes in the patient's
environments (hospitalization, bereavement point out a marked difficulty in
adjustment abilities. When seen in office examination, the patient's
complaints are vague and they tend to rely on notes or other aids to memory.
A curious lack of concern and flattening of affect may alternate with periods
of transient depression early in the illnesses. On testing, the patients
show global deficits in orientation and memory but recent memory is affected
in a more severe fashion than immediate and remote memory functions. In
this context, a simplified 'mini-mental state' examination has been
developed by Folstein, Folstein and McHugh[21]. The validity of this examination has been well documented. It is simple, reproducible and easily
administered in the course of a general evaluation. In earlier and middle
stages of senile or pre-senile dementia, the remainder of the neurological
examination is within normal limits and the general physical findings are
not contributory. Further laboratory examination should include lumbar

puncture with cerebrospinal fluid evaluation. (If normal pressure hydrocephalus is suspected from the history and physical findings, this examination
should be deferred to the time of radionuclide scanning). It is noteworthy
that SCF protein measurements tend to be low in senile dementia. Blood
studies should include folate, cyanocobalamine levels and tests of thyroid
hormone function. Electroencephalography is less valuable in diagnosis
since non-specific diffuse slow activity is usually the only abnormality
discernable. Skull X-rays per se are not useful and pneumoencephalography
to demonstrate ventricular dilation has been superceded by the introduction of
computerized axial tomography (CAT scanning) since the early seventies. This
technique involves neither risk nor discomfort for the patient and CAT
scanning perhaps is the laboratory study of greatest importance in senile
dementia.

Although the most useful laboratory method, CAT scanning
is not without pitfalls. Early in the disease when diagnosis may be difficult,
the X-ray findings of brain atrophy do not correlate well with clinical
findings[22]. Radionuclide scanning to monitor transependymal flow of cerebrospinal fluid is essential to exclude brain atrophy secondary to hydrocephalus
(normal pressure hydrocephalus). Utilizing radioactive Xenon cerebral blood
flow can be combined with CAT scanning to evaluate a vascular component in
patients with senile change[23, 24]. For the future positron emission tomography
(PET)[25] promises to be the major tool for regional evaluation of the brain.

In summary, senile or pre-senile dementia is a disorder
of major social and economic importance. Each case demands most careful
attention by the clinician. Since there is no effective treatment for
dementia associated with senile brain atrophy, it is essential that remedial
causes of dementia be recognized early and effective treatment promptly
started. It should be noted that treatable cases can range from ten to
twenty percent[17, 18] of all patients with behavioral change and suspect

dementia. Despite major advances in radiological techniques, the diagnoses are clinical and ultimately dependent on historical review, and on mental and physical examination findings.

REFERENCES:

1. The Aging Veteran (Oct. 1977) Present and Future Medical Needs, Veterans Administration report, 89.
2. Webster's Third New International Dictionary (1971) Gove Pub G&C Merriam Co., Springfield, MA. p. 477
3. DeLong, N., Russell,   (1967) The Neurologic Examination 3rd Edition Hoeber Medical Division, Harper & Row Pub. New York, Evanston and London, 38.
4. Paulson, G.W. (1971) in Dementia Wells, C.E., ed. Contemporary Neurology Series. F.A. Davis Pub., Philadelphia, p. 13-33
5. Teuber, H.L. (1950) in Recent Advances in Diagnostic Psychological Testing Harrower, M.R., ed. Charles C. Thomas Pub., Springfield, Ill, pp. 49-72
6. (a) Obrist, W.D. (1954) EEG & Clin. Neurophysiol., 6, 235.
   (b) Fridlander, W.J. (1958) 13, 29.
7. Weiner, H. and Shuster, D.B. (1956) EEG & Clin. Neurophysiol., 8, 479.
8. Oldendorf, W.H. (1961) IRE Trans. Biomed. Electronics (BME) 8, 68.
9. Hounsfield, G.N. (1973) Brit. J. Radiol. 46, 1016.
10. Kistler, J.P., Hochberg, F.H., Brooks, B.R., Richardson, E.P., New, P.F.J. and Schnur, J. (1975) Neurol., 25, 201.
11. Barron, S.A., Jacobs, L. and Kinkel, W.R. (1976) Neurol., 26, 1011.
12. Gado, M.H., Coleman, R.E., Lee, K.S., Mikhael, M.A., Alderson, P.O. and Archer, C.R. (1976) Neurol. 26, 555.
13. Hodkinson, H.M. (1977) Biochemical Diagnosis of the Elderly, John Wiley & Sons Pub., NY, pp. 28-34
14. Wells, C.E. (1978) (a) Psychiatric Annals, 8, 58.
    (b) ibid. Amer. Psych. 135, 1.
15. Freeneon, F.R. (1976) Arch. Neurol., 33, 658.
16. Marsden, C.D. and Harrison, M.D.C. (1972) Brit. Med. J. 2, 249.
17. Victoratos, G.C. and Herzberg, L. (1970) Brit. J. Psychiat., 130, 131.
18. Smith, J.S., Kiloh, L.G., Ratnavale, G.S. and Grant, D.A. (1976) Med. J. Australia 2, 403.
19. Seltzer, B. and Frazier, S.H. (1977) in the Harvard Guide to Modern Psychiatry. A.M. ıholi, Jr., ed. Harvard University Press, Cambridge, MA, pp. 297-318.
20. Seltzer, B. and Sherwin, I. (1978) Am. J. Psychiat., 135, 13.
21. Folstein, M., Folstein, S. and McHugh, P. (1975) J. Psychiat. Res. 12, 189.
22. Fox, J.H., Topel, J. L., Huckman, M.S. (1975) Geriatrics, 30, 97-100.

Published 1979 by Elsevier North Holland, Inc.
Nandy, Ed. Geriatric Psychopharmacology

SLEEP AND AGING

MILTON KRAMER, M.D., DIRECTOR, DREAM-SLEEP LABORATORY, VETERANS ADMINISTRATION
HOSPITAL, CINCINNATI, OHIO AND PROFESSOR OF PSYCHIATRY, UNIVERSITY OF CINCIN-
NATI, CINCINNATI, OHIO

The modern scientific resurgence of interest in sleep has taken place over
the past 25 years[1]. Since the observations of Kleitman, Aserinsky and Dement
that isolated so called "dreaming sleep", there has been a significant alteration in our fundamental understanding of the organization of the sleep state
and the processes which occur during sleep[2].

It had long been assumed that sleep could be understood as simply the absence of wakefulness. Essentially, this point of view argued that sleep was a
geared down wakefulness. Sleep was, then, to be understood as wakefulness
minus, an absence state.

Sleep is best conceptualized as a state which is differently organized than
wakefulness. This is, perhaps, best illustrated by the alterations which occur
during the REM portion of sleep. The EEG becomes more like wakefulness, the
basic autonomic functions of respiration, blood pressure and heart rate become
highly irregular and mental content is dream-like. This state which recurrent-
ly occupies some 20-25 percent of adult sleep is not more or less wakefulness,
but different than the wakefulness state[3].

A frequent corallary of the view of sleep as an absence state is that sleep
is a passive process. It is captured in the idea of falling asleep rather than
going to sleep.

It is clear from the research evidence that sleep is an active process during which events occur at rates both different from and sometimes greater than
wakefulness. For example, some neuron groups are firing at rates higher than

during wakefulness. Although not fully elucidated, the sleep onset process is probably a function of active mechanisms rather than just a gearing down of an active process. And, the alterations within the sleep state are clearly under the control of active processes, e.g. those that initiate and control REM state[4].

A third aspect of the traditional view of sleep, the first is that sleep is an absence state and the second is that sleep is a passive state, is that sleep is <u>unitary</u>. This is a view that sees two basic states of the organism, wakefulness and sleep, and further sees sleep as all of a whole, i.e. all hours of sleep are the same.

It has become abundantly clear that sleep is not a unitary state. Sleep is organized into two basic states, NREM and REM, which alternate throughout the night. Further, the NREM state can be effectively divided into substates which have been labeled as sleep stages (I, II, III, IV) which also tend to be sequentially organized within the NREM state.

There is supporting evidence to suggest that significant biological phenomenon systematically co-vary with the various subdivisions of sleep. This provides the legitimizing biological rationale for these distinctions within sleep. For example, NREM sleep is associated with serotonin mechanisms while REM sleep has been found to relate more to changes in nor-epinephrine. NREM sleep, particularly stages III and IV, is related to growth hormone release. Night terror-nightmare, somnambulism and enuresis are related to NREM sleep, particularly to arousals from it. REM sleep, as has been noted, is related to cardio-respiratory irregularities, dream-like mental content and suggestively to brain protein alteration. Stages of NREM sleep reflect an increasing arousal threshold, supporting an ordered relationship along a sleep depth continuum [5,6,7].

Sleep, then, is not an empty (absence), passive, unitary state. Rather, sleep is a uniquely organized, active, multifaceted state.

From a functional point of view, sleep has other attributes of great interest. Sleep is both variable (responsive) and stable. Sleep is maleable but not infinitely so.

Sleep is responsive to drugs[8], the social context[9], illness[10] and crucially for our present purposes, aging[11]. There is a wide range of pharmacological agents that affect sleep either by lengthening it, shortening it or altering its internal architecture. The social context in which sleep occurs affects its onset, maintenance and concurrent mental content, i.e. dream content. Disease, both psychiatric like depression, anxiety neurosis and schizophrenia can affect sleep; and physical disease, such as hypo and hyperthyroidism, asthma and pain related illnesses as well. Some illnesses are thought to be actual disturbances of the sleep system, i.e. nocturnal myoclonus, narcolepsy and hypersomnia with periodic apnea (HPA)[12,13,14,15]. And, as we will discuss, aging itself appears to play havoc with the integrity of sleep[16].

Despite the responsivity of sleep to many factors some of which like drugs, social context, disease and aging were enumerated above, sleep in both its physiological and psychological components is a relatively stable process. Sleep is not an infinitely manipulable function[17]. It has been pointed out that sleep will respond to its deprivation by becoming finally preemptory. Sleep, viewed as a need, is more like respiration than it is like hunger or sexual desire. Sleep cannot be indefinitely postponed.

Sleep has a rather regular and predictable pattern in its occurrence. This is the case both physiologically and psychologically[9]. On a night to night basis, one nights sleep does, indeed, predict the next nights sleep. This is equally true for both the physiological parameters of sleep, e.g. total sleep time, time in stage REM sleep, and psychological parameters, e.g. number and type of characters present in the sleepers dreams.

Sleep is a uniquely organized, active and multifaceted state which is both variable and stable. The central role of this biological activity, sleep, in the adaptive processes of the individual is intuitively apparent but unsuccessfully demonstrated scientifically. Nevertheless, an examination of the significant alterations of sleep in the aging process seems worthwhile.

CLINICAL SLEEP PATHOLOGY

It has long been recognized that one of the major bodily processes which alters as a function of aging is sleep[11]. It has even been suggested that changes in sleep might well serve as an index not just of the aging process, but of the maturational process as a whole[16,18].

In aged persons, concern about the reduction in the hours of sleep and complaints related to sleep are disturbingly common. It has been estimated that some 15 to 30 percent of Americans complain about their sleep. And, that some 9 million not only complain, but have used sleeping pills nightly for a least one year to attempt to enhance sleep[19]. Such sleep complaints and medication use are even more wide spread in older people.

Now it is necessary to take serious alterations in hours of sleep, complaints about sleep and the accompanying medication used[20]. All of these factors have been found to co-vary negatively with longevity. It is not that sleep alterations cause death, but that sleep is a bodily function that is highly sensitive to pathological disturbance. Disturbed sleepers are, from a mortality point of view, a high risk group.

It can no longer be said with complete impunity that sleep is an individual matter. If you get four hours of sleep and feel and function up to your satisfaction, there still is beginning grounds for concern. There is evidence to suggest that there is an optimum amount of sleep a person should be getting.

It has been shown that the number of hours of sleep an individual reports as typical for him co-varies with longevity. Independent of any report of sleep complaint, individuals who report sleeping eight hours a night have a lower death rate over the next six years than those who report a shorter or longer sleep period. Further, as the deviation from the proverbial eight hours increases, either less than eight or more than eight, the mortality rate increases. At four hours or less for men or ten hours or more for women, the risk of death within six years is about the same as it would be if the individual had hypertension, diabetes, a stroke or coronary artery disease.

Further, it has been observed that those who complain of problems with disturbed sleep have an increase of 20 to 30 percent in mortality rates. Problems with disturbed sleep, so common in the aged, reflect a decreased capacity for survival.

The common treatment for sleep disturbance is a hypnotic drug. Once these are started, they are very likely to be continued. Frequent sleeping pill use enhances the mortality risk some 50 percent. The sleep disturbance provides a modest risk increase which our common treatment apparently doesn't correct but appears to enhance.

In the older person, sleep and its complaints need to be taken seriously. Sleep itself is sensitive to the aging process. Alterations in the hours of sleep, intensified with aging, are related to an increased mortality rate. Complaints related to the disruption of sleep also are more common in older people. And lastly, sleeping pill use which even more intensely than hours of sleep or sleep disturbance increases mortality rates are more frequently used in older people. Sleep is clearly a legitimate and important focus of medical attention in aged person.

THE SLEEP ELECTROENCEPHALOGRAM

The cyclic alteration of NREM-REM across the night (sleep period) about every 90 minutes, with stage I to stage IV changes occurring in the NREM phase has already been described. The so-called deepest stages of sleep, namely III and IV, occur early in the night and stage REM occurs later in the night.

Each stage of sleep can be characterized by the presence and quality of eye movements, the level of muscle tone measured at the neck and nature and special features of the EEG[21]. Stage wake has sharp eye movements, a high level of neck muscle tone and an alpha rhythm on the EEG. Stage I has slow rolling eye movements, a high level neck electromyogram and theta and vertex waves on the EEG. Stages II, III and IV have no eye movements, high level muscle tone and are differentiated based on the EEG. Stage II has spindles and K-complexes, stage III has 20-50 percent delta waves and stage IV, 50 percent delta waves or more. REM stage has sharp eye movements, low muscle tone and a low voltage mixed frequency fast EEG with saw-toothed waves.

From a developmental point of view, one may characterize the changes in sleep as a function of age as resulting in more time awake and less time spent in NREM sleep[11]. When looked at a bit more strictly, there is an increase of wakefulness with a severe loss of deep sleep and a more modest loss of REM sleep.

Data provided from normal sleepers between ages 3 and 79 illustrates the maturational process. Time spent in bed goes down but then rises again in old age, while the time spent asleep goes down and rises just a bit in old age. The aged spend more time in bed but do not really get more sleep. If one looks at wakefulness, it increases with age gradually but abruptly increases in old age. Older people do, indeed, spend more time awake. Both stages III and IV and REM sleep are decreased in old age. The REM decline is gradual while the stage III and IV decline is more abrupt.

There is clearly a change in sleep associated with maturational processes with marked changes occurring in old age. The increased amount of wakefulness and increased number of arousals described by aged sleepers does reflect their biological experience. Some have said it indexes the aging process. However, explanations of the process are not forthcoming. It is of some moment that men show sleep changes about ten years before women do, perhaps a reflection of the differential aging process known to exist between the sexes.

DREAMS AND THE AGING PROCESS

There are both biological and psychological aspects to aging as there are to sleep. Some of the biological changes in sleep with aging have already been reviewed. In the present section, the effects of aging on dreaming will be explored by examining the dream recall rates and dream content of aged person.

Dream recall from REM period awakenings in the laboratory is between 75 and 85 percent and is only modestly age dependent. There is more of a suggestion that recall is sex dependent with women recalling more dreams than men. However, in aged populations, there is reason to believe that there is a decrease in dream recall and that both the aging process and organic changes in the brain contribute to the decline in recall, the latter more than the former[22].

It has been reported that 50 year old men with mild organic brain damage recalled dreams from 57 percent of awakenings while in those with severe organicity the recall percentage was 35 percent. In contrast, 70 year old men with milder organicity had a recall percentage of 79 percent while those with severe organicity recalled dreams from only 8 percent of awakenings.

These recall rates set the limits to the study of dream content in aged populations. Little material is available to the dreamer and very few studies have been directed to exploring the dream life of older people.

In the survey of normative dream content[23], it was also found that individuals 65 or older reported fewer dreams than younger people. Older people are more concerned with death and destruction (death anxiety and death themes) than younger people. Younger people are concerned about guilt while aged individuals are much less so.

It has been pointed out that dreams can be vehicles to understand the dreamer. Certainly, the content of the dreams of aged persons point to their concern with the end, with death. This, perhaps, becomes, if confirmed, a depar-
ture point for understanding the older person.

It may be a value to note the effect of organicity on dream content. More
organically damaged patients as compared to age and sex matched less organic
ones have more characters in their dreams. Will the older person who confronts
the loneliness of death respond as do the more brain damaged with an increase
in the number of characters in their dreams? Will this be related to people
seeking behavior on the part of the older persons?

The inner processes of the aged remain to be explored. The examination of
dreams may help us to understand the older person as it has to some degree
younger people.

HYPNOTIC DRUGS IN THE AGED

It has already been pointed out that the aged have clear alterations in
sleep and attendant complaints about their sleep. Aged persons complain particularly about difficulty initiating and maintaining sleep and not feeling re-
freshed after sleep. They are the premier example of the triad of insomniac
complaints. Older people use and are prescribed more hypnotic medication than
other age groups although the safety and effectiveness of such an approach has
been questioned.

Literature on the effects of drugs on sleep, although extensive, suffers
from major shortcomings. It is, therefore, difficult to feel confident about
the pharmacological solution to sleep disturbances in insomniacs in general and
in geriatric insomniacs in particular.

A review of the literature reveals its limitations[24]. While two thirds of
the studies of the effect of drugs on sleep have been done in the sleep

laboratory, where more careful monitoring is possible, only 60 percent were of
hypnotic drugs. The laboratory studies examined only very few subjects in each
experiment and, typically, studied the drug effect for only one night. This is
not useful when we realize that most insomniacs have used sleeping pills nightly for a year or more.. These laboratory studies did in 66 percent of the cases
examine more than one dose of a drug, while the larger non-laboratory studies
only examined more than one dose of a drug 20 percent of the time. Most dis-
heartening has been the lack of attention to the systematic examination of side
effects in studying the effects of drugs on sleep. Only one third of the studies reviewed systematically report side effects. This is clearly an insufficient number especially for this class of drugs whose primary effect at one
point in time, within the same subject, becomes a side effect in another, i.e.
sleepiness.

Most limiting for our understanding of the role of hypnotics in geriatric
patients is the small number of studies exploring the effects of these hypnotics in geriatric patients. Although they are, or will be, one of the major
target populations for any hypnotic drug, only 3 percent of the studies have
utilized older subjects. The absence of laboratory exploration of hypnotic
drug effectiveness in aged populations is even more striking.

It has been suggested that the failure of an early non-laboratory study to
show discriminability among hypnotic agents, although it did show an active
drug-placebo difference, coupled with the stringency of FDA regulations has
discouraged the study of hypnotic drug effectiveness in older populations. It
might be useful to illustrate the drug-placebo and drug-drug differences can be
shown using hypnotic agents in an aged population even utilizing a questionnaire as the instrument of inquiry[25].

Chloral hydrate 250 mgs and 500 mgs were compared to the effects of a new
triazalo-benzodiazepine (triazolam) in .25 and .50 mgs doses and to a placebo.

The test population was a group of 25 insomniac men, over the age of 65, resident in a nursing home. Further, the patients estimate of sleep duration showed that triazolam 0.5 mgs produced significantly longer sleep estimates than chloral hydrate 500 mgs. The data showed that for sleep onset and for number of awakenings, triazolam 0.50 mgs produced significantly faster sleep onset and a smaller number of awakenings than placebo or chloral hydrate 500 mgs. Finally, the quality of sleep was reported to be best with triazolam 0.50 mgs. It may be concluded that a post-sleep questionnaire is sensitive to differences between drug and placebo as well as between two drugs.

The careful assessment of hypnotic drug efficacy and safety in laboratory and non-laboratory studies in geriatric populations is both necessary and possible. Without such a systematic undertaking, the effective treatment of sleep disturbances in insomniac geriatrics will not be possible.

CONCLUSIONS

Sleep is clearly altered in older people in potentially damaging directions. Aged persons spend more time in bed, do not sleep more and have more time awake. They have less stage IV and less REM sleep. People over 65 recall fewer dreams and those they do recall have a greater concern with death and destruction and less guilt than those of younger people.

Hypnotic drug studies in aged populations are few in number and suffer from being non-laboratory and studying too few subjects, for too few nights at too few doses of drug and with insufficient systematic reporting of side effects. Laboratory and non-laboratory studies of hypnotic efficacy and safety in geriatric populations is both feasible and desirable.

REFERENCES

1. Webb, W. B. (1973) Sleep: An Active Process, Research and Commentary. Glenview, IL: Scott, Foresman and Company.
2. Dement, W. C. (1972) Some Must Watch While Some Must Sleep. Stanford, CA: Stanford Alumni Association.
3. Kramer, M. (1969) Paradoxical Sleep. Postgrad. Med. 45:157-161.
4. Hobson, J. A. and McCarley, R. W. (1977) The Brain as a Dream State Generator: An Activation-Synthesis Hypothesis of the Dream Process. Am. J. Psychiat. 134:1335-1348.
5. Hartmann, E. (1978) The Sleeping Pill. Boston, MA: Yale University.
6. Cartwright, R. D. (1978) A Primer on Sleep and Dreaming. Phillipines: Addison-Wesley.
7. Weitzmann, E. D. (1974) Advances in Sleep Research, Volume I. Flushing, NY: Spectrum Publications, Inc.
8. Williams, R. L. and Karacan, I. (1976) Pharmacology of Sleep. New York, NY: John Wiley and Sons, Inc.
9. Kramer, M. and Roth, T. (In Press) The Stability and Variability of Dreaming. Sleep.
10. Kales, A. (1969) Sleep Physiology and Pathology-A Symposium. Philadelphia, PA: J. B. Lippincott Company.
11. Williams, R. L., Karacan, I. and Hursch, C. J. (1974) EEG of Human Sleep, Clinical Applications. New York, NY: John Wiley and Sons, Inc.
12. Zorick, F., Roth, T., Salis, P., Kramer, M. and Lutz, T. (1978) Insomnia and Excessive Daytime Sleepiness as Presenting Symptoms in Nocturnal Myoclonus. Sleep Res. 7:256.
13. Guilleminault, C., Dement, W. C. and Passouant, P. (1976) Narcolepsy. Holliswood, NY: Spectrum Publication, Inc.
14. Lugaresi, E., Coccagna, G. and Mantovani, M. (1978) Hypersomnia with Periodic Apneas. Jamaica, NY: Spectrum Publications, Inc.
15. Guilleminault, C. and Dement, W. C. (1978) Sleep Apnea Syndromes. New York, NY: Alan R. Liss, Inc.
16. Feinberg, I. (1976) Functional Implications of Changes in Sleep Physiology with Age. Neurobiol. of Aging, pp. 23-41.
17. Webb. W. B. (1975) Sleep, The Gentle Tyrant. Englewood Cliffs, NJ: Prentice Hall, Inc.
18. Roffward, H., Muzio, J. and Dement, W. (1966) Ontogenetic Development of the Human Sleep-Dream Cycle. Sci. 152:604-619.
19. Karacan, I., Thornby, J., Anch, M., Holzer, C., Warheit, G., Schwab, J. and Williams, R. (1976) Prevalence of Sleep Disturbance in a Primarily Urban Florida County. Soc. Sci. and Med. 10:239-244.
20. Kripke, D. F. (1979) Short and Long Sleep and Sleeping Pills. Arch. of Gen. Psychiat. 36:103-116.
21. Rechtschaffen, A and Kales, A. (1968) A Manual of Standardized Terminology Techniques and Scoring System for Sleep Stages of Human Subjects. UCLA Brain Information Services.
22. Kramer, M. and Roth, T. (1975) Dreams and Dementia: A Laboratory Exploration of Dream Recall and Dream Content in Chronic Brain Syndrome Patients. Int'l. J. Aging and Human Development 6:169-177.
23. Winget, C., Kramer, M. and Whitman, R. M. (1972) Dreams and Demography. Canad. Psychiat. Assoc. J. 17:203-207.
24. Roth, T., Kramer, M. and Salis, P. (In Press) Drugs, REM Sleep and Dreams. Handbook of Dreams: Research, Theory and Applications, Wolman, B., Ullman, M. and Webb, W. B. (eds.).
25. Roth, T., Kramer, M., Felson, J., Grissom, T. and Lutz, T. (1976) Evaluation of Hypnotics in Geriatric Patients. Sleep Res. 5:77.

Published 1979 by Elsevier North Holland, Inc.
Nandy, Ed. Geriatric Psychopharmacology

TREATMENT OF COMMON PSYCHIATRIC DISORDER IN THE ELDERLY

KENNETH NOBEL, M.D.
Department of Psychiatry, Harvard Medical School, Boston, Massachusetts

INTRODUCTION

This chapter will discuss the management of common psychiatric syndromes of
elderly people, emphasizing modifications which need to be made in order to
adapt standard therapies to the special needs of the elderly. In general, drugs
which are effective for younger patients are equally effective for older ones.
Indications for pharmacologic intervention may, however, look different since
common psychiatric illness may present in unusual ways in old people. Dosage
schedules often need to be changed from those to which we are most accustomed.
Equally important, the entire clinical interaction, of which the administration
of an appropriate drug in the appropriate dosage is only a part, needs to be
modified. Normal aging involves considerable physiological and psychological
flux, in many ways similar to the well recognized upheavals of adolescence at
the other end of the span of years we call adulthood. This flux and its
attendant emotional reactions must be accounted for in managing the illnesses
of old age, especially the psychiatric conditions. For these reasons, considerable attention will be devoted to the overall therapeutic approach to the
various syndromes to be discussed as well as to the clinical context in which
medications are administered. Only by combining appropriate pharmacologic
treatment with an appropriate interpersonal relationship can we offer our
elderly patients the best possible care.

A GENERAL APPROACH TO THE PATIENT WITH DISORDERED BEHAVIOR

The initial presentation of an elderly patient with psychiatric illness is
often chaotic. Frequently there are associated physical symptoms and/or medical
illnesses. The patient himself may not perceive the problem as an emotional
one and may resist treatment and see the clinician as a threat. Family, friends
and even physicians may also not recognize a psychiatric illness for what it
is until all supportive resources are exhausted, so that these patients frequently present in crisis. Even without a crisis situation the elderly patient
may be so far removed from the invariably younger clinician in background,
education, outlook and values, that he is as culturally alien as someone from
another country. Elderly people are especially sensitive to their emotional
surroundings and often the first therapeutic agent. Specially effective in

this regard is the presence of a clinician who is able to act calmly, to make sense of the problem, and to offer some hope of assistance.

For all of these reasons, the first efforts in management must be directed specifically at establishing a therapeutic alliance. The clinician must communicate explicitly his interest and concern, help to generate a climate of trust and understanding, and work to establish mutually relevant goals. This should be an active process with two not necessarily sequential components. First, there must be a clinical negotiation in which the patient is encouraged to state as explicitly as possible his own perception of the problem, his initial expectations of the therapeutic interaction and his fears about it. The clinician may then respond directly to concerns which might otherwise be left unspoken and which could sabotage the entire treatment plan if not explicitly addressed.[1] For instance, many depressed patients assume without discussion that "senility" is part of their problem, are mortally afraid of electro-convulsive therapy (E.C.T.), or hold idiosyncratic beliefs about drugs. Unless these kinds of issues are actively looked for and discussed the first sign that clinician and patient hold different understandings of the therapeutic process may be noncompliance with a drug regimen or inclusion of the clinician in a paranoid system.

Second, the clinician must work to communicate as concretely as possible his interest in the patient as a person and not only in the disordered behavior. With younger patients this empathy is communicated by a variety of relatively subtle, nonverbal cues which might be missed or misinterpreted by an older person who is likely to have at least minor sensory deficits in addition to being infirm, frightened, alienated and sometimes confused. With elderly people, a number of simple modifications in technique serve to increase the sense of contact and empathy. In general, these modifications tend in the direction of making the interaction more immediate, more comprehensible and more explicitly focused on real life issues meaningful to the patient: 1) It is usually advisable to sit closer to an elderly patient and to maintain eye contact actively, insuring that clinician and patient can both hear and cutting down the real estrangement often felt by the elderly. 2) Physical contact, a friendly squeeze of the hand or pat on the shoulder is often appropriate as a concrete expression of interest and understanding, although personal and cultural mores must be kept in mind and respected. 3) Whenever possible, the language of the interaction should be that to which the patient is accustomed; the language customarily used to describe feeling states is somewhat foreign to many old people. 4) It is often helpful for the clinician to make himself less alien and mysterious by sharing more of his own life and experiences than he might with a younger patient. 5) Direct advice is often more appropriate than traditional interpretive techniques. Psychiatric symptoms frequently arise in response to real life problems which have overwhelmed coping strategies that the patient is not likely to be able or willing to change through the achievement of insight. 6) In almost all cases, it is essential to work not only with the patient but with the family and other caretaking people as well. Optimal management may not be possible without their involvement, and they can often offer essential historical information as well.

Another important understanding which helps in relating appropriately to elderly people is to recognize the special place of the past in their lives. One of the important developmental tasks of old age is to come to terms with the accumulated experience and achievements (or lack of them) of a lifetime, and from this to build a sense of completion, acceptance and, hopefully, satisfaction.[2] An important source of self-esteem for old people is a recognition, particularly by younger people, of the interest and value of their life experiences. One corollary to this is that it is very important for a clinician to pay special attention to the past history of his elderly patients. This will provide essential information regarding characteristic coping styles, strengths and vulnerabilities, and will also allow an opportunity to recognize, support and validate an important source of self-esteem for the patient. Exploration of the past with an older person is an important cornerstone of treatment, and should not be considered "wandering" or inappropriate.

Along with these adjustments in technique, it is important to modify the goals of therapeutic intervention when working with elderly psychiatric patients. A simplistic model where the expected outcome is cure, or eradication of a discrete pathological process, is rarely appropriate, and such an expectation will only lead to frustration and excessive pessimism on the part of both patient and clinician. A more realistic goal in most cases is management and stabilization of a process which is likely to require care on an ongoing, or at least recurrent basis. Likewise, to expect major personality changes from an elderly patient, is not realistic. The psychological focus of normal old age is much more on preservation of previously acquired adaptive skills than on change or growth, in the usual psychological sense. The efforts of the helping clinician are most appropriately directed towards conflict resolution, towards helping to mobilize previously successful defenses and coping strategies and adapting them to the problems of old age. Since people respond to the problems of old age in a very individual manner, goals of intervention need to be individualized, explicit and tailored to the patient's needs rather than to the clinician's preconceived notions of what ought to be accomplished.

DEPRESSION

   Depression in elderly people is characterized by an increased prominence of the somatic components of the depressive syndrome and by apathy, withdrawal, and poorly focused anxiety with relatively little of the usual depressive effect. The patient may appear hypochondriacal or bland and disinterested rather than depressed. Disability is frequently perceived as being due to normal aging, senility or physical illness. There is often resistance to accepting a psychiatric diagnosis manifested in part by vigorous insistence on another explanation. All of this makes diagnosis difficult and interferes with treatment once the diagnosis is established. Nevertheless, most depressions in elderly people respond very well to appropriate treatment, and age should be no barrier to therapeutic optimism or endeavor.[3]

   An approach to the depressed elderly patient begins with the formulation that in their old age many people are deprived of important sources of "narcissistic supplies"--they lose contact with experiences and people who help them feel worthwhile, safe, loved and cared for.[4] In many cases it is the lack of these narcissistic supplies more than the existence of loss, guilt and self-directed anger which contributes to the development of depressive states. It follows, therefore, that therapeutic maneuvers designed to help to establish a feeling of personal safety and security, to recover a sense of being a valuable and worthwhile person, and to remember that he is (or has been) loved and cared for by others, are especially important for the elderly patient. An excellent first step is to support and encourage discussion about the past, since this is an important source of self-esteem in old age. For a younger professional person to be interested in his past life and willing to listen to stories about it helps an elderly patient to re-establish his own connection with his past and its value. It might be added that virtually every older person has something in his past which he considers valuable. Even people who have made masochistic adaptations to life or who would appear to have achieved very little can point with some pride to having survived and can usually find sparks of warmth, strength and comfort where superficially we would see none.

   Another important source of well being for the elderly is their social network which is usually disrupted or strained by a depressive illness. Sometimes it is a change or strain in the social network which precipitates the depression but often this is a secondary phenomenon. A knowledgeable, supportive,

realistic, nonjudgemental clinician can help to keep families and other people
engaged by helping to establish reasonable expectations and correct misconceptions about the depressive illness. Where conflict or guilt exists, this can
be worked through with the care-taking people to help restore nuturing relationships and break up destructive ones. Reasonable limits on behavior can be
worked out which will allow increased comfort for all concerned. Finally,
simply helping a depressed older person to identify his realistic needs and
then to meet them within the growing network of social service agencies may
help to lift a depression in the absence of any other treatment. A homemaker,
meals on wheels, or extra disability income may help to restore a sense of
personal security and serve as a powerful antidote to depression. The need
for such services should be looked for quite specifically since people may be
embarrassed to ask or may accept deprivation as their appropriate state and not
connect these needs to how bad they feel. It is not enough to identify the
need for services; the providers may need some professional support in dealing
with an elderly client who may appear cantankerous and difficult, especially at
first.

More traditional psycho-therapeutic interventions may also be useful in
dealing with grief or with situational conflicts. The goal of such intervention
is support, conflict resolution and mobilization of defenses which may have
been overwhelmed or undervalued. With this approach clinicians frequently find
that they have much to offer their older patients.

Although interpersonal interventions can sometimes substitute for drug
therapy and always supplement it, the fact is that most older depressed patients
require pharmacologic intervention. Typical neurovegetative signs occur as an
indication for drug treatment. Appetite disturbance may be especially dramatic
and cognitive slowing can occur to the point that it mimics a dementia. The
mainstay of pharmaco-therapy, as in younger patients, is the tricyclic group of
antidepressants. Most evidence indicates that these drugs are as effective in
the elderly as they are in younger people. Dosages, however, must be modified
to account for slower absorption, metabolism and excretion in elderly people.
In general, only one-third to one-half of the usual dose is required to attain
therapeutic blood levels, 30-100 mg. a day of Imipramine or Amitriptyline or
equivalent doses of other drugs.[5] The lower doses are appropriate for smaller
and frailer people. It should be borne in mind, however, that there is much
more biological variability among the elderly compared to younger populations.
Some older people may tolerate and require full doses of tricyclics to obtain
a therapeutic benefit. Another consequence of the slower biological handling
of the drugs in old people is that a steady state equilibrium in the blood is

achieved more slowly and onset of drug action may take as long as six weeks.[5]
Because oversedation is a particular problem in old people the less sedating
Imipramine group of drugs is usually preferable. Because it has the lowest
level of anticholinergic activity of the Imipramine derivatives, Desipramine is
probably the drug of first choice. One drawback to the use of Despiramine,
however, is that it is not currently formulated in 10 mg. tablets, so that
modulating the low recommended doses is sometimes impossible. Where agitation
or sleeplessness are especially prominent, one of the Amitriptyline group of
drugs is indicated, again in doses starting at one-half to one-third of the
usual adult range.

As with all medical interventions in the elderly, side effects can be
particularly troubling. Toxicities which may appear minor in younger people
can cause serious disability in the elderly. Oversedation and lethargy are
frequent. Toxic delirium may occur. Anticholinergic effects may include
urinary retention, particularly in men, and this should be specifically looked
for because patients may be embarrassed to mention it. Constipation may be
precipitated or made worse, causing physical discomfort which is magnified by
the depressed state. Dry mouth, although rarely serious, is nearly universal.

It is especially important to be aware of possible cardiovascular side
effects of tricyclic antidepressants. The commonest of these is orthostatic
hypotension, a drop in blood pressure when going from supine to sitting or
sitting to standing positions which occurs in both young and old patients. It
is less well tolerated in elderly people and can lead to syncope, to falls, or
in extreme cases to compromised perfusion of vital organs. It is therefore
essential to follow sitting and standing blood pressures frequently, especially
when treatment is first instituted and to inquire specifically for the presence
of light headedness on rising or with exercise. There is much concern regarding
direct toxic effects of tricyclics on the myocardium, precipitated by reports
claiming an excess of sudden death in patients treated with Amitriptyline[6] and
by the recognition that people dying of tricyclic overdoses have ventricular
arrhythmias refractory to treatment. The excessive incidence of sudden death,
has, however, been convincingly disputed in another study[7] and the relevance
of effects of excessive dosages to every day clinical practice would seem to
be questionable. There are also data which suggest a Quinidine-like effect on
the heart and prolonged AV conduction[8,9] but clinical correlations of these
observations are lacking. Certainly there is ample reason to believe that
Tricyclics have some potential for cardio-toxicity, but this is true of many
drugs such as Digitalis, Quinidine, and Propranolol which are prescribed every
day in medical practice. It would seem most reasonable at the present time to

screen elderly patients with an electrocardiogram (EKG), to follow them closely for orthostatic hypotension and irregularity of the pulse and to be alert for symptoms which suggest syncope. It is easy and convenient to spend a few minutes on each visit feeling the radial pulse, which is very useful for detecting arrhythmias and may also provide the kind of concrete expression of interest and concern required to break through depressive isolation. Patients with high degrees of heart block or periods of ventricular irritability should be treated cautiously, followed even more closely and perhaps considered sooner for E.C.T. instead of drugs. If, however, there are clear neurovegetative signs of depression, the coexistence of cardiac disease should be considered an indication for caution and the exercise of clinical judgement but should not be an absolute contraindication to treatment.

MAO inhibitors are seldom used in this country because of their potential for cardiovascular side effects and the dietary restrictions which need to accompany their use. They are, however, used in Britain and Europe and might be considered if tricyclics are ineffective or cannot be used and if proper dietary compliance can be assured. Electroconvulsive therapy is both safe and effective in the elderly and allows the opportunity for closer monitoring of the patient's cardiovascular status before and after each treatment. Post-ECT confusional states may be more severe in the elderly, so that hospital observation is usually preferable.

Lithium is indicated in elderly people for bipolar manic depressive illness, and sometimes, for a recurrent unipolar depression. As with tricyclics, therapeutic blood levels can be attained with low doses in most, but not all, cases.[10] A reasonable initial dose would be 150 mgs. twice a day with a slow increase as indicated to achieve blood levels between 0.8 and 1.2. As always with Lithium therapy, renal function, thyroid function, and electrolyte status should be followed along with Lithium levels. A fine tremor is a common side effect, but is usually not disabling. Gastrointestinal toxicity can be minimized by taking the drug with meals. Toxic confusion is, as always with the elderly, a serious potential problem. Administration of a phenothiazine along with Lithium, as is often done in acute mania, may induce toxic confusion, not reproducible by administration of either drug alone, so that combination therapy should be avoided if possible.

PSYCHOSIS

This discussion will focus on the psychotic states which arise for the first time in old age, so called late life paraphrenias or involutional psychoses. The symptoms of these psychoses of late life tend to be relatively circumscribed compared to the generalized systems of autistic thinking seen in schizophrenia. Often there is a single, intensely held, fixed delusion whose content is less bizarre and more immediate than a schizophrenic delusion. From the point of view of management, what is most important is that, unlike schizophrenia, the content of the delusional material is often directly related to a real life conflict or problem. The delusion serves to project and deny the conflict, which would otherwise be overwhelming to the ego. Often, delusional thinking serves to restore self esteem where it has been threatened or to mitigate losses, including loss of status or function. The content of the delusion serves as a "clue" to the precipitating problem, allowing the clinician access to conflict-ual material not otherwise accessible. Picking up this clue allows for more accurate reality testing and more appropriate supportive interventions. For example, an elderly, deaf widow living alone developed the delusion that a neighbor was talking about her and was playing a radio to torment her. The neighbor, had, in fact, been rude which added to the many narcissitic injuries the patient had suffered by reason of age and infirmity. Attempts by family to deny the reality of the delusions produced only anger and frustration. Recognizing the real situation allowed the patient to ventilate appropriate anger towards the neighbor and to re-establish herself in her own eyes as "better" than the neighbor. The need for the delusion was therefore less and it became much less insistent.

Among the problems which may precipitate psychosis in the elderly is physical illness. A biological derangement may impair brain function or the illness may imply a threat of suffering, disability and death which is overwhelming for the patient. Another important precipitant of psychosis is dementia and it may be psychotic symptoms which first bring a dementing patient to medical attention. Sensory deficits may also be associated with psychotic symptoms. In all these cases the psychosis may be conceptualized as a desperate attempt to bring some order to a situation which is incomprehensible and frightening and to mobilize some help from what appears to be an unresponsive environment. The patient may deny or minimize the underlying real life problems, focusing instead on his psychotic defensive maneuvers. It follows, therefore, that special attention must be paid to assessing the intellectual and sensory capacities and the medical status of an elderly psychotic patient. A careful search should also be made for social problems, losses, and changes in important relationships which may have precipitated the psychotic state. Once identified, these can be addressed realistically and supportively, thereby reducing the need for the psychosis.

It is also important to work with family and caretakers who often are bewildered by psychotic symptoms and either become angry and withdraw or engage in futile efforts to contradict the patient's delusional beliefs. If they can be helped to deal realistically with the underlying reality issues, to reduce expectations the patient can not meet (for instance, that he always makes sense when he speaks) and to take over activities the patient can not realistically perform, they become vital therapeutic allies. For instance, if an elderly person is convinced that he is being robbed by the bank, help with the check-book is more appropriate than a flat denial of the delusion which the patient is unlikely to believe; it is important for a clinician to help the family see this and to respond appropriately. Work with the patient can then focus on supporting him accepting appropriate help and on rebuilding self esteem. As with all psychotic patients communication must be clear, simple, and unambiguous and consistent limits must be set.

Psychotic symptoms in the elderly may be transient, responding quickly to supportive measures, reality testing and environmental manipulations as dis-cussed above. Delusional beliefs may persist but not be acted on or responded to. In these cases, no pharmacologic intervention is necessary. Antipsychotic drugs are indicated when delusions are acted on and responded to with inappro-priate behavior, when sleep is consistently disrupted or when there is uncon-trollable anxiety. The anxiety may be manifested as frantic help-seeking behavior such as calls to the police or to the family to come and set things right. Anxiety may also be entirely unfocused leading to generalized panic with a virtual dissolution of personality and of intrapsychic defenses.

The usual antipsychotic agents are very useful in controlling psychotic symptoms in the elderly. It is not clear that any one of them is especially effective and the choice of a drug should be made on the basis of which the expected side effects would be most dangerous to the patient. Since the most disabling side effect is usually lethargy, the less sedating drugs such as Haloperidol, Trifluoperazine, Acetophenazine or Perphenazine are usually preferred. There is increased risk of extrapyramidal side effects with these drugs but in low doses this is usually not disabling. If there is a greal deal of agitation or if there is a gait disturbance, Thiroidazine might be used first, since it is more sedating and has relatively few extrapyramidal side effects. Stronger sedatives, such as Chlorpromazine, should be used with extreme caution, if at all.

Doses of all antipsychotic drugs should be kept small in comparison with the usual adult doses. Effective symptom control can be achieved with 0.5-6 mgs. of Haloperidol, 2-10 mgs. of Trifluoperazine, or 25-300 mgs. of Thioridazine in

24 hours, or with equivalent doses of other drugs. In most cases it is reasonable to expect a reduction in anxiety and somewhat more realistic thinking in a few days. If there is no improvement, the dose of medication may be increased slowly until there is improvement or toxicity precludes further increases. It may be necessary to supplement low initial doses with "extra" doses on a PRN basis for episodic agitation, especially in the first few days of treatment.

The most disabling side effect of antipsychotic drugs is, as already stated, mental slowing and lethargy. Since the drugs are long acting, blood levels may be expected to rise for a week or even longer, so that a drug which appears well tolerated after a few days may cause lethargy after several weeks. This is not necessarily an indication to stop treatment. Often holding the medication for a few days and resuming at a lower dose maintains effective symptom control without excessive side effects. When assessing a lethargic patient, care should be taken to distinguish mental slowing from paucity of movement or slurred speech due to a movement disorder. Sometimes patients with dementia and psychosis appear to decline intellectually with drug treatment. In some cases this apparent decline may not be due to drug side effect, but to unmasking of the dementia as the psychosis improves and is not, therefore, an indication to modify treatment. Because of this possibility, it is important to pursue a thorough assessment of the intellectual capacity of every psychotic elderly patient.

In the very low recommended doses extrapyramidal side effects are usually not a serious problem, though they can, of course, occur and should be watched for. Akathesias may be mistaken for agitation if not specifically considered. Acute dystonias and parkinson-like syndromes usually respond to appropriate antiparkinsonian medication. The incidence of extrapyramidal side effects is sufficiently low, however, that routine administration of antiparkinsonian drugs, which have their own risk of central nervous system toxicity, is not advisable. The elderly are especially susceptible to tardive dyskinesias and should be carefully watched for buccolingual movements. Since it appears that this complication is, to some extent, dose related,[11] this serves as another argument for the use of low doses of antipsychotic drugs in the elderly.

Like antidepressants, antipsychotic agents may have cardiovascular toxicity. Usually the toxicity takes the form of orthostatic hypotension, although there are a few reports of myocardial toxicity and of significant arrhythmias.[12] Thioridazine is most often associated with arrhythmias,[13] though other drugs have also been implicated. As with antidepressants, it is important to monitor the pulse, as well as sitting and standing blood pressures, although hypotension

is usually less of a problem with antipsychotic drugs than with tricyclic antidepressants.

In general, the less sedating drugs (piprazines, butyrephenones) are more
likely to cause extrapyramidal side effects and the more sedating ones are more
likely to be associated with cardiac and anticholinergic side effects. Anticholinergic side effects may include urinary retention, especially in men. This
can usually be treated with small doses of Bethanechol (Urecholine, 10-20- mgs.
q.i.d.) and are not an absolute indication to stop antipsychotic drug therapy.

ANXIETY

Anxiety in old people can often be linked to specific problems and dealt
with by counseling or supportive psychotherapeutic techniques as previously
discussed. It may also be relieved by assessing and meeting realistic needs
or services. When such interventions alone are not sufficient to reduce symptoms
or when the patient is dysfunctional because of anxiety, drug treatment is
indicated.

The effectiveness of antipsychotic drugs for anxiety associated with
psychosis has been discussed. Clinical experience suggests that the same kind
of disorganized pan-anxiety or panic very often occurs without an associated
breakdown of reality testing in elderly people, especially those who are more
debilitated physically and/or mentally. Rather than experiencing their anxiety
as a symptom outside themselves, they are overwhelmed by it, are unable to
elaborate any psychological defenses against it, and appear to undergo a dissolution of personality and intellect under the pressure of their anxiety. It
appears most reasonable to treat such people with antipsychotic medications,
even though they are not formally psychotic. If, on the other hand, the
patient's coping capacities and personality structure remain intact, if he is
able to see the anxiety as a circumscribed problem outside himself, if he is
more intact physically and mentally, then treatment with a benzodiazepine antianxiety agent would seem more reasonable.

Benzodiazepines are demonstrably effective in controlling symptoms of
anxiety in the elderly,[14] but must be used with caution because their long
half-life allows slow build up to toxic levels. While the shorter acting drugs,
such as Lorazepam or Oxazepam, would seem to offer theoretical advantages in
this regard, no conclusive clinical evidence exists to allow a recommendation of
one benzodiazepin over another. Over-sedation is the most worrisome side effect
of these drugs. These drugs should be prescribed at one-half to one-third of
the usual adult dose for elderly patients.

Many elderly people have literally grown old with the barbiturates and feel that they benefit from their use. Objectively, however, there is no reason to prefer barbiturates over benzodiazepines for anxiety control. Their strong sedative effect, interference with hepatic metabolism of drugs, and addiction potential make the barbiturates less desirable overall than either benzodiazepins or phenothiazines.

REFERENCES

1. Lazare, A., et al. (1975) Arch. Gen. Psychiat., 32, 443.
2. Butler, R.N. (1963) Psychiatry, 26, 65.
3. Epstein, L. (1976) J. Gerontol., 31, 278.
4. Zinberg, N., and Kaufman, I., (Eds.) In, Normal Psychology of the Aging Process. (1963) New York, International Universities Press.
5. Nies, A., et al. (1977) Am. J. Psychiatry, 134, 790.
6. Coull, D.C., et al. (1970) Lancet, 2, 590.
7. Swett, C.P., and Shader, R.I. (1977) Dis. Nerv. Syst., 38, 69.
8. Bigger, J.T., et al. (1977) N. Engl. J. Med., 296, 206.
9. Burckhardt, D., et al. (1978) J. Amer. Med. Assoc., 239, 213.
10. Hewick, D.S., et al. (1977) Brit. J. Clin. Pharmacol., 4, 201.
11. Crane, G., and Smeets, M. (1974) Arch. Gen. Psychiat., 30, 341.
12. Hollister, L.E., and Kosek, J.C. (1968) J. Amer. Med. Assoc., 205, 108.
13. Giles, T.D., and Modlin, J.K. (1968) J. Amer. Med. Assoc., 205, 108.
14. Salzman, C., et al. (1975) J. Amer. Geriatrics. Soc., 23, 451.

POLYPHARMACY AND DRUG-DRUG INTERACTIONS IN THE ELDERLY

CARL SALZMAN, M.D.
Associate Professor of Psychiatry, Harvard Medical School, Massachusetts
Mental Health Center, 74 Fenwood Road, Boston, Massachusetts 02115

Elderly users of psychotropic drugs take drugs in combination more often
than do users of other prescription drugs.[1] In surveys of medical practice in
general hospitals and nursing homes, it was found that older patients tend to
receive an average of five to twelve medications every day.[2]   Psychotropic
drugs are likely to be mixed with other psychotropic drugs.[3,4] In a survey of
elderly patients in 12 Veterans Administration hospitals, eighteen percent received two or more psychotropic active drugs. However, 77 percent of patients
received ten or more drugs when nonpsychiatric drugs were included.[5] Tracy and
Shader (cited by Salzman, 1975)[6] surveyed polypharmacy in three distinct populations: 87 healthy non-institutionalized volunteer research subjects; 337
residents of several nursing homes around the Boston metropolitan area; and 136
inpatients of a psychiatric hospital. Common drug combinations included
psychotropic drugs with sedative-hypnotics (48.4% of drug combinations) with
diuretics (24%) and with antihistamines (7-14%).

Salzman has recently surveyed elderly inpatients on general hospital medical-surgical services and has extended these previous data.[7,8] 32.7 percent
of patients over the age of 60 were taking psychotropic drugs. Table 1 lists
the categories of most frequent drugs prescribed. The mean number of drugs
taken was 8. Table 2 illustrates the average list of drugs taken on the survey day by a patient who received a psychotropic medication.

TABLE 1

CATEGORIES OF MOST FREQUENTLY PRESCRIBED DRUGS

Psychoactive

      Flurazepam
      Other sleep medications
      Neuroleptics (phenothiazines and butyrophenones)
      Tricyclic antidepressants
      Antianxiety (primarily diazepam)

Medical

      Non-narcotic analgesia (e.g., ASA and acetominophen)
      Narcotics
      Antibacterials
      Additives (Vitamins, Fe SO_4, KCL, etc.)
      GI elimination (DOSS*, MOM)
      Cardiovascular (Digoxin, quinidine, antihypertensive)
      Antihistamine

*Dioctyl sodium sulfosuccinate (Colace and Pericolace); Milk of Magnesia

TABLE 2

AVERAGE ELDERLY PATIENT TAKES EIGHT DRUGS

      Flurazepam
      ASA or Acetominophen
      MOM
      Anti-bacterial
      Dioctyl Sodium Sulfosuccinate
      Diazepam
      Propoxyphene
      Vitamins

Polypharmacy lists were developed from the survey data to illustrate geriatric polypharmacy and prescribing practices in a general hospital. Tables 3 to 6 list the 7 average drugs taken with the index psychotropic medication which were prescribed to nearly all elderly patients. The tables suggest an overall similarity of polypharmacy drug prescription. The lists, of course, may be reversed. A patient taking digoxin, meperidine or DOSS is likely to be taking the same 7 drugs with nearly interchangeable psychotropic medication. Thus for elderly general hospital patients on these medical-surgical services, it is possible to predict with some confidence how many and what type of drugs each will be getting. In turn, this allows for an anticipation of high probability drug-drug interaction which may be clinically useful as well as toxic.

TABLE 3

SEVEN DRUGS MOST FREQUENTLY TAKEN WITH FLURAZEPAM* (in decreasing frequency)

Digoxin
DOSS or MOM
ASA of acetominophen
Meperidine or Morphine
Vitamins, KCL, Ferrous Sulphate or Gluconate
Antibiotic
Diphenhydramine or Prednisone

*Flurazepam was the most frequently prescribed drug.

TABLE 4

SEVEN DRUGS MOST FREQUENTLY TAKEN WITH DIAZEPAM* (in decreasing frequency)

DOSS or MOM
Digoxin
ASA or acetominophen
Meperidine or Morphine
Antibiotic
Vitamins, KCL, Ferrous Gluconate or Succinate
Diphenhydramine or Prednisone

*Diazepam was the most frequently prescribed non-hypnotic psychotropic drug; with the exception of one chlordiazepoxide prescription, it was the exclusive antianxiety drug prescribed.

TABLE 5

SEVEN DRUGS TAKEN MOST FREQUENTLY WITH TRICYCLIC ANTIDEPRESSANTS (in decreasing frequency)

Digoxin
Antibiotic
Vitamins, KCL, Ferrous Gluconate
DOSS or MOM
ASA or Acetominophen
Meperidine or Morphine
Neuroleptic

120

TABLE 6

SEVEN DRUGS TAKEN MOST FREQUENTLY WITH NEUROLEPTIC DRUGS* (in decreasing
frequency)

ASA or Acetominophen
DOSS or MOM
Vitamins, KCL or Ferrous Gluconate
Meperidine or Morphine
Digoxin
Diphenhydramine
Antibiotic

---

*Antinausea phenothiazines, primarily prochlorperazine, are included in this
list because of similar drug-drug toxicity to neuroleptics.

The most common examples of clinically useful drug-drug interactions in general hospital patients is the enhancement of sedation or analgesia (Table 7).
Neuroleptics or benzodiazepines (most frequently diazepam) are most often combined with other CNS sedatives to quiet the agitated elderly patient. Agitation in the elderly may be post surgical, secondary to disorientation in an
intensive care unit, due to organic brain syndrome related behavior, or a consequence of drug toxicity.

TABLE 7

FREQUENTLY USED DRUG COMBINATIONS IN A GENERAL HOSPITAL ELDERLY POPULATION*

Desired Effect	Clinical Indication	Psychotropic Drug Used	Drug Combination
1. Sleep	Insomnia likely in elderly; worse in unfamiliar surroundings or when anxious as in a hospital	Flurazepam	Often combined with other CNS sedatives, analgesics, and sedating psychotropic drugs
2. Daytime sedation	Agitation, post surgical confusion, precarious medical condition	Diazepam Chlorpromazine Thioridazine Amitriptyline	Often combined with narcotic analgesics, nighttime sedatives
3. Anti-anxiety	Anxiety is common in elderly with declining health and support systems	Diazepam almost routinely prescribed in hospital survey; other benzodiazepines having limited use	Often combined with analgesics
4. Anti-agitation	Toxic confusion, OBS	Haloperidol Thioridazine Chlorpromazine	Often combined with other CNS sedatives and analgesics

*This list reflects actual frequency count rather than a recommended list of drug combinations.

Elderly patients in a general hospital are also likely to be treated for severe pain which may result from disease such as cancer or from surgery. Neuroleptic drugs, such as haloperidol, chlorpromazine and thioridazine, are often combined with narcotics to augment CNS sedation and analgesia. When nausea is a prominent symptom, prochlorpromazine is often used. Since this is a piperazine side chain phenothiazine, it too can augment the CNS depressing analgesic effect of narcotics.

Unwanted psychotropic medical drug interactions in the elderly general hospital patient most commonly fall into one of three categories: 1) oversedation (CNS underarousal), 2) anticholinergic effects, and 3) toxic cardiovascular effects (Table 8). The combination of sedating psychotropic drugs such as neuroleptics, benzodiazepines or hypnotics with other CNS depressants, such as narcotics, may produce an unwanted side effect of CNS sedation.

TABLE 8

UNWANTED CLINICAL EFFECTS OF DRUG COMBINATIONS

Unwanted Effects	Psychotropic Drug Used	Drug Combination
1. Over sedation	Neuroleptics Benzodiazepines Amitriptyline Doxepin	Sedative-hypnotics, narcotics, analgesics, cytotoxic substances, antihypertensive medications
2. Anticholinergic effects	Neuroleptics Tricyclic antidepressants	Narcotics, atropine containing drugs, antihistamines
3. Cardiotoxicity	Tricyclic antidepressants	Combined with antihypertensives, antiarrhythmics

Elderly patients with depressed CNS functioning are more sensitive to the disorientation produced by CNS underarousal than are younger patients. This is particularly true in the evening and at night (Sundowner's Syndrome) when orienting perceptual stimuli are decreased. The behavioral result is often confusion, agitation and irritability. Elderly general hospital inpatients, who may already be disoriented and who are CNS underaroused, sometimes try to climb out of bed, mistake nurses for family members, have frightening periods of amnesia, or may even hallucinate. A typical medical response is to add more sedating drugs, particularly neuroleptics, which either further aggravates the clinical situation or puts the patient to sleep.

The same combination of neuroleptic and narcotic drugs, along with tricy-clic antidepressants, is also responsible for heightened anticholinergic effects. The elderly patient, particularly those with organic brain dysfunc-tion are particularly susceptible to these effects.[9-11] Patients develop severe dry mouth (and may lose porcelain dental fillings) and an increase in urinary stasis. Constipation, which is often already present in the elderly and particularly in older general hospital patients, becomes severe. Consti-pation may be the symptom which produces the most discomfort in the older patient and which makes him increasingly irascible and uncooperative. The CNS consequences of anticholinergic drug activity, however, are most likely to pro-duce unwanted cognitive and behavioral side effects. Older patients easily become confused, disoriented and hallucinatory. Toxic hallucinosis, worse at night, may encourage erroneous medical diagnoses (e.g., cancer metastases to brain or rapid onset organic brain deterioration). The patient becomes less cooperative, more irritable and even combative. As families and nursing per-sonnel become alarmed, the patient is prescribed another psychotropic drug with anticholinergic properties, often a neuroleptic. One elderly patient in the general hospital survey who was thought to be depressed following surgery was prescribed amitriptyline in addition to the thioridazine already prescribed for augmentation of sedation and analgesia. As she grew increasingly restless, the doses of both psychotropic drugs were increased. Amitriptyline was finally discontinued when the patient began to hallucinate, and the symptoms cleared in two days.

Unwanted cardiovascular side effects of psychotropic-medical drug interac-tions are particularly hazardous in the elderly, especially if there is heart disease. These interactions, however, are less frequent than the two discussed

above. Enhanced quinidine-like effect may result from the addition of tricyclic antidepressants to quinidine preparations. Enhanced hypotension may
result when tricyclic antidepressants are combined with antihypertensives.
The well known interaction between tricyclic antidepressants and guanethidine
drugs, while hazardous, is unlikely: no patients in the general hospital survey received such a combination. Similarly, the toxic consequences of MAO
inhibitors in elderly hospitalized patients taking cardiovascular medications
is serious, but unlikely. No elderly patients were taking MAO inhibitors at
the time of the survey.

The survey data suggest that other well known psychiatric drug-medical drug
interactions while potentially serious are also unlikely. The combined use of
antacids with benzodiazepines or other drugs was relatively infrequent (only 7
of 62 elderly patients received antacids). No patient received steroids,
estrogens or thyroid in combination with antidepressants. The use of enzyme
inducing drugs such as barbiturates was infrequent (two elderly patients
received pentobarbital, one received phenobarbital).

On the basis of the surveys of psychotropic drug use and polypharmacy in
elderly populations, it is possible to formulate several generalizations regarding psychotropic drugs and polypharmacy in the elderly.

1. Psychotropic drugs including sedative-hypnotics are frequently com-
    bined with non-psychotropic drugs. This is true for normal elderly,
    elderly research volunteers, and geriatric medical patients. Drugs
    which are most frequently combined with psychotropics are cardiovascular
    medications, analgesics and laxatives.

2. Elderly residents of nursing homes and VA hospitals, both medical and

psychiatric, are more likely to have combinations of two or more psychotropic drugs given simultaneously than normal elderly, or elderly medical inpatients. This may reflect a higher age patient group, or a selection of patients whose cognition and behavior is so severely disordered
that they cannot live in a non-residential facility.

3. Combinations of psychotropic drugs are more common in long-term care
psychiatric facilities than in short-term general hospitals. Such combinations, however, may produce severe CNS toxicity, particularly in the
patient who is already CNS underaroused, confused or disoriented.

4. Polypharmacy as a routine practice may be hazardous. Therapeutic drug
combinations, which affect CNS arousal states or cholinergic function
are most likely to produce unwanted toxic reactions. In order to reduce potentially toxic drug-drug interactions unnecessary psychotropic
medications should be avoided. Patients need not be routinely given
sleep medications or antianxiety agents. Sadness may be appropriate to
the clinical situation and not a symptom of clinical depression which
requires antidepressant treatment. Agitation in the elderly may be a
consequence of polypharmacy or OBS as well as a symptom of emotional
distress.

REFERENCES

1. Guttmann, D. (1978) in Medication Management and Education of the Elderly,
    Beber, C.R. and Lamy, P.P. ed., Excerpta Medica, Washington, pp. 18-19.
2. Kalchthaler, T., Coccaro, E. and Lichtige, S. (1977) J. Am. Geriatr. Soc. 25,
    308-313.
3. Fracchia, J., Sheppard, C. and Merlis, S. (1971) J. Am. Geriatr. Soc. 19, 301-
    307.
4. Fracchia, J., Sheppard, C., Canale, D., Ruest, E., Cambria, E. and
    Merlis, S. (1974) J. Am. Geriatr. Soc. 11, 508-511.
5. Prien, R.F. (1975) in Aging, Volume 2, Gershon, S. and Raskin, A. ed.,
    Raven, New York, pp. 143-154.
6. Salzman, C., Shader, R.I., and Harmatz, J.S. (1975) in Aging, Volume 2,
    Gershon, S., and Raskin, A. ed., Raven, New York, pp. 259-272.
7. Salzman, C., and van der Kolk, B.A. (1979), submitted for publication.
8. Salzman, C., and van der Kolk, B.A. (1979), submitted for publication.

9. Salzman, C., Shader, R.I., and Pearlman, M. (1970) in Psychotropic Drug
    Side Effects, Shader, R.I. ed., Williams and Wilkins, Baltimore, pp. 261-
    279.
10. Salzman, C., van der Kolk, B.A., and Shader, R.I. (1975) in A Manual of
    Psychiatric Therapeutics, Shader, R.I. ed., Little,Brown & Co., Boston,
    pp. 171-184.
11. Salzman, C., Shader, R.I., and van der Kolk, B.A. (1976), N.Y. State J.
    Med. 76:71-77.

DEPRESSION, DEPLETION AND DEMENTIA: A RATIONAL BASE FOR
A COMPREHENSIVE THERAPEUTIC APPROACH TO A SPECIFIC CONDITION
OF LONG-LIVED PEOPLE

STANLEY H. CATH, M.D.
Medical Director, Family Advisory Service and Treatment Center,
Inc., 18 Moore Street, Belmont, MA 02178

An unusual man, famous in our field, lived a very long and
creative life. His output continued through two world wars, sur-
viving the Nazi scourge as well as a migration to a new land. His
work developed into one of the major influences of all time upon
almost all men. Very often, modern writers, attempting to stand
on this man's shoulders, claim to see even further on the horizon,
or to dare criticize him for what he did not see three quarters of
a century ago. In regard to the former, this author is no exception. I, too, would like to see further than Freud, but what I
have to say is but a small addition to his ideas. Let me begin by
quoting a lead of his relative to my thesis. Despairing after
some 30 operations for cancer of the jaw, this famous if contro-
versial man, feeling his life was ebbing, wrote to Marie Bonaparte,
"My situation is a small island of pain floating on an ocean of indifference." He also observed, "To someone else, my diagnosis
would be depression."[1] As I reflected on this distinction and synthesized my clinical work with the elderly with his self observations, I realized my diagnosis of Freud at that time would not be
depression, either. Rather it was depletion-depression and the
complex fluctuating relationship between these two conditions. In[2]

128

my judgement, all seven life styles* of people in the last trimes-
ter of life are never just depressed. They struggle with new forms
of age specific anxieties, with new fluctuations in intensity of
affects in a series of new human discomforts of both organic and
psychological origins. Aging changes are inwardly sensed along
with perceptions of changes in basic resources or in the "background of safety."[3] The challenge of a long life is to maintain a
constant sense of self in a changing body and a changing world.The
passage of time, then, always includes elements of continual organic change of variants of psycho-social-physiological depletion as
well as depression. It is a time of loss, mourning and attempts
at creative restitution. At times like these, significant others
are of tremendous value. In all but the most severely demented,a
physician should never say to an individual or family that there
is nothing medicine can do and then abandon them. Rather, the physician can recognize and utilize his limited assets, recognize the
needs of the elder and his more youthful family and capitalize on
the refueling power created by the human need for relationships
and basic attachments. On occasions, he can indeed reverse organic biochemical end-products of stress, the so called reversible
dementias, but even in intractable cases, he can treat the depressive factors and tendencies for depletion in all basic anchorages
wherever possible. Even in moderately severe dementias, maintaining as healthy a state of nutrition, well being and attachment
as possible will depend upon recognizing that there is, indeed,

---
*
  1. hysteric, 2. obsessive 3. inadequate 4. depressive
  5. dependent, 6. paranoid 7. schizoid

a mourning process in progress in almost every long-lived human being and his loved ones. This is possible even in moderate to severe dementia, almost to the end. While acknowledging our igno- rance and relative impotence to ourselves, our patients and the family, keeping hope alive is something that can be done. In my opinion, it is our responsibility to do this, to maintain hope, as we study the varieties of human responses to the rupture of attachments made over a lifespan and to the loss of intactness in the ideal self-other world.

I. Depression

"He is a fool that is not melancholy once a day." (Old Russian Proverb)

Depression is essentially a change in mood, subjectively cha- racterized by varying feelings of sadness, helplessness, hopeless- ness, and worthlessness. There is a lack of joy which effects the way in which the individual perceives himself and the world around. It may be accompanied by anxious agitation and by somatic symptoms such as headaches, ab- dominal pain, fatigue, constipa- tion and sleep disturbances.

In the struggle to understand and classify there has been considerable ambiguity about this most commonly diagnosed pheno- menon in the world, namely, that of depression. Some believe as the proverb expresses, that it is a part of normal living from day to day. Others that it is an uncertain disease of non-homo- geneous nature of which no satisfactory systematic classification has yet been devised. We do not completely understand when ordi- nary sadness converts into more serious neurotic depression, when it becomes psychotic or circular and why spontaneous or seemingly miraculous remissions occur. To illustrate the degree of our en- lightenment in 200 years we have come full circle. In the seventeenth century this syndrome was described as circular. As modern scientists we use the word bi-polar.

Thus, depression covers two phenomena at least. The first, one of the two daily life-long normal core affects involved in the response to loss of or threats to attachments (anxiety and depression) and the second, a pathological phenomenon of being down in mood, a clinical condition usually lasting for a self limited time.

I have come to consider late-life depression as a disease extending beyond ordinary degrees of despair, disillusionment, disgust, demoralization, dejection, dysphoria, despondency and defeat. I will submit, with advancing years, still another phenomenon is added to reach a new level of complexity. This addenda consists of the very real process of normal depletion and its associated age specific task of mastering "depletion anxiety". This syndrome complex when added to various degrees of pre-mid-life helplessness and hopelessness constitutes a new psycho-social physical entity 'depression-depletion'. But it is a complex still reversible (up to a point) by a combination of psycho-social-physiological approaches. It may be because of gerontophobic reactions by physicians to its complexity that depression-depletion plus the onset of dementia takes on a generally regarded irreversible prognosis to a condition previously considered reversible by psychotherapy, emotional refueling, sleep deprivation, drugs, electric shock therapy, and environmental manipulations.

Thus, we come to a series of ponderous but related questions the answers to which are only partially discernable. Is depression an inevitable accompaniment of decreasing activity, vitality and productivity of all aging organisms or only of particularly

vulnerable ones? My hope is to illustrate how the total internal
and external environment "the ego ecological system" is crucial in
universally depressive depleting syndromes. Let me be the first,
however, to acknowledge that depression is virtually unknown
among many cultures i.e. the natives of equatorial Africa whose
life span is 40-50 years, but I must also note that depletion is
universal and present there. Cultures which become westernized almost invariably show an increase in numbers of people subject to
affective disturbances. Is depression an intrinsic part of an
organic aging process related to changes in biochemistry i.e. increased levels of MAO in the brain? It certainly is the most
common world wide psychiatric diagnosis as noted above. Still only five percent over age 65 have a well defined classical depression.[4] Is depression the same all throughout the life span?
Roughly, it has been observed from ages 8-80. According to Spitz[5]
in his study of "Hospitalism", i.e. infants experience an "anaclytic depression". My experience inclines the answer towards the
negative. Depression is not the same through a lifetime even if
the same kinds of defenses against threats to attachments are
triggered and/or the same kinds of chemical changes can be documented i.e. one could prove that 50 percent of depressives hyper-
secrete cortisol from 8-80. A person is not the same ego-ecological organism at 65, at 35 or at eight months. Furthermore, a depression may first occur in latency or in the postpartum period
or very late in life, in the 60's or 70's. Once again, I believe
depression-depletion takes place in a differently structured,dif-
ferently reservoired and differentially aging human being. The
next question is: is depression in the form of sadness, grieving

or mourning adaptive? and is it not more destructive in the worst
forms of melancholy with suicidal fixation? I believe depression
is different in each set of circumstances. For some, it represents
a mislearned, early in life, once-adaptive phenomenon, an anachro-
nism of withdrawal and retardation in the present but still ex-
pressing that the fantasied loss of attachment will be corrected.
An analogy might be hibernation or the anaclytic depression of
infants. For others late in life it is different and represents
a crescendo or omniconvergence of accumulated real loss and
change.[6] It even may eventuate because the resiliency of the ego
and the supporting ego-ecological system is less capable of ward-
ing off or of coping with ravages of altered psycho-physiological
states. This may be due to exhaustion of vital chemical elements,
or with the death of a spouse or supporting other, of vital narcissistic supplies which influence chemical-immune mechanisms. Replacement of vital objects, if possible, alters feedback of vitalizing input into the system. Still there may be one set of psy-
cho biochemical conditions at one point in one cohort of depressives and another set at another. All of this leads me to ask
have we really known what depression is, how many forms are there
of it and have we ever appreciated its complexity? I think it is
a syndrome people have recognized historically and cared for heu-
ristically in different cultures along very similar lines,namely
as a disordered response to the threat of or actual rupture in
caring attachments. In Japan 'Morita therapy' assigns one person to a patient to gratify basic needs. In the west, cases
where external events were visibly involved in triggering the attack, i.e. the death or fantasied death of a loved one or one upon

whom one was unusually dependent, i.e. long lived couples, it has been traditional for depression to be called exogenous or reactive. In other cases, when the person seemed in poor contact with reality, when low mood is associated with delusions or no trigger was evident, depression might be considered a more severe pathological disorder and referred to as endogenous. Others defined depression as primary or secondary and preferred to think in terms of "affective disorders". But you may know the latest change (DSM-3) maintains affects are transitory and moods more permanent. Accordingly, we may soon discard affective disorders for a classification of mood disorders, major and minor. In an apparent attempt to simplify the picture, the major will be divided into uni-polar and bi-polar. Unfortunately, recent research suggests that bi-polars may have different genetic roots or genetically are heterogeneous.

Theorists range from those who believe depression is a true neuro-endocrine disturbance to those psychoanalytic thinkers whose conceptual emphasis i.e. on empathic failure leads to the impression they are not thinking around an organic or instinctual base. As early as 1925, Freud[7] said, "The ego is first and foremost a body ego" and eventually we must look for answers to bio-chemistry. Today no matter what school one belongs to, any scientific thinker must acknowledge and take into consideration bio-chemical markers for depressed states which reflect important bio-chemical disturbances. Research has especially focussed our suspicions upon increased norepinephrine, serotonin and dopamine in the neuro transmitter system. Discrete urinary factors such as altered MHPG levels are considered to reflect, among other things, the hyper-secretion of cortisol, derived ultimately from a dis-

turbance in catecholomines at the neurotransmitter junctions. Cortisol levels seem to be sensitive to changing phases of depression.
But under stress, one loses the usual circadian rhythm and cortisol rises.   If one gives a normal patient diximethosone as a cortisol suppressant, the cortisol level drops to zero in 24-36 hours.
In a depressed patient it may also decrease but it will rebound
quickly: i.e. if given at 8:00 a.m., the level will rebound by
4:00 p.m. Via this technique, we can differentiate 50 percent of
depressions as supposedly endogenous but 50 percent do not show
this rebound.   Some think a faulty HPA axis (the hypothalamic pituitary adrenal axis) may be involved, in that biology of depression
suggests an individual is all revved up.   With a reasonably intact
nervous system depressed people seem to be spinning their wheels
internally.   Heart rate and breathing can be increased or may be
irregular.   A redistribution of cations led to studies of membrane
physiology and the electrochemical differences in ordinary well
being and depression.   In later years, an increased monaminoxidase
level is found in the hind brain as well as in higher level neuro
transmitter junctions.   But endocrine researchers tell us this
level is inversely related to estrogens, that is, the lower the
estrogens, the more the monoamineoxidase.   These observations are
reinforced because a disturbance in the hypothalamic-pituitary
thyroid axis is reflected by an increase in free thyroxine.   Thus,
major depressive disease raises many questions having to do with
important neuro-regulatory endocrine centers.   But these, in
turn, also seem to relate to circadian rhythms.   Is it as simple
as one theory which suggests   that there is a failure to turn
off the hyper-secretion of cortisol at night and that the norepi-

nephrine levels mirror or are a mirror image of the circadian cortisol phenomenon. Is this just a disturbance of circadian rhythm
or is sleep architecture at the root of this complicated disease;
or is the crucial factor the pleasure centers of the brain which
seem out of whack.[7] This leads to the impression the most common
denominator in major depressive diseases has been suggested to be
the lack of ability to enjoy pleasure either in the past or future.
It is to see the self as helplessly enmeshed,hopelessly, in a set
of circumstances out of which the only desirable end may seem to
be a cessation of living.

On the basis of the evidence presented so far, that is, the
endocrine neuro-chemical base or disordered cerebral centers, attempts to change chemistry and/or shift the recall of unpleasant
memories or convictions based on conscious images and gestalts
have been made and all are part of the more usual therapeutic re-
gimes. These include a range of psycho-tropic drugs, psychother-
apies and various other forms of treatment i.e. electro-shock and
sleep deprivation. Still not all psychiatrists can agree either
on the diagnosis, prognosis or treatment plan for any specific
constellation or syndrome. Feeling therapy must be as complex
and comprehensive as the disease, itself, I will proceed to add
still another complication.

II. Depletion as an Organic Factor in Human
Late-life Adaptability

While we may consider paradigms as beacons which guide us in
understanding health and disease, we must acknowledge they are limited by our conceptual language. Even in physicians, such language more often than not is colored by individual and collective

motivation, education, social values and psychological tendencies.
I still would venture to suggest four paradigmatic beacons in medicine: the natural or genetic, the biological or organic, the family and/or sociological and finally the psychological or meaningful purposes of life. All physicians are biased by their own coefficient of anxiety and select one of those paradigms which seem
most critical to them for heuristic or theoretical purposes. While
I, too, would like to believe in the ancient notion nature heals
and destroys in her own wisdom, it seems to me that medicine can
never assume that nature is above needing a little help. The late
natural history and continuing integrity of a family will depend
to a great degree on the paradigms, attitudes and wisdom of the
physician as well as those of the scientific community around him.
Intervention and better understanding may come from a number of
sources and disciplines to influence this balance. Let me give
an example.

Many years ago a social worker, learning of my work with the
elderly, decided although she lived in San Francisco, to request
a consultation for her father. Over the past two years, he had
been seen and evaluated by local physicians who considered his
slow progressive decline in cognitive, social and personal skills
were due to hardening of the arteries, for which nothing could be
done. From an inventive, intelligent, spontaneous man with a lo-
ving sense of humor, he became withdrawn, a shadow in the background
of family affairs. For the most part he showed little initiative
except for family gatherings. Although he complained of his arthritis, otherwise he did not seem too unhappy or in pain. At family gatherings, he pulled himself together trying very hard to do

the right thing. In fact at these times, he seemed his old self.
This confused the family who thought he was pretending or just
asking for attention by his confusion or lack of participation at
other times. With most of his social graces intact, he would
often shop with his wife, but major decisions were no longer in
his hands and the family learned not to ask him for important decisions. He seemed to care little about this shift in status. For
no apparent reason, he had fallen on two occasions. My evaluation
revealed a still charming, pleasant and interesting man with much
recent and intermediate memory loss especially about current events
in his world. Strong evidence of spatial impairment, and rather
poor drawings of a house, flowerpot and clock suggested considerable right frontal hemisphere damage. My cursory physical examination including a superficial neurological were essentially normal, as in the past. I decided on a mild cerebral stimulant
which especially facilitates neuro transmission, an antidepressant and some vitamins as a psychopharmacologic regime. Then I
spent considerable time with him and his family reviewing the circumstances and what might be happening. I covered depletion as a
natural aspect of aging, I suggested there are unknown immune factors which also deplete or are exhausted so a virus may cause a
certain number of brain cells to function intermittently. By cal-
ling on all his reserves, I could explain there were times he was
his old self. But these cells were exhausted easily, especially
if vital supplies were limited, one could not expect him to function at the steady level they had been accustomed to in the past.
If his condition were not too severe, possibly we could tip the
scales a little and some improvement might be possible. At least

we would try. Within the short time of a week, his condition improved sufficiently so that both he and his family were extremely
pleased. He called Hydergine his "pain killer". In retrospect
he regarded our visit about which he had been initially quite concerned, as quite pleasant. Because of the episodes of confusion
and falling, I thought it best to investigate more thoroughly,
the possibilities of TIAs, and he was ready to accept a referral
to a West Coast geriatric psychiatrist to do this and for follow
up care. During the course of the examination by this supposedly
sophisticated colleague, the patient asked, "What do you think is
wrong with me". The colleague's answer: "You tell me what's
wrong with you". After completing his examination he turned his
back to the family and said, "I don't know what's wrong with him.
What do you want me to do?" Truly confused, they said, "Well, Dr.
Cath thought you would do a more thorough examination and see if
there is anything more that can be done." (I had thought of anti-
coagulants or aspirin to try reducing clotting tendencies if
TIAs were, indeed, the problem). This doctor shrugged his shoulders and said, "He has a progressive,organic deterioration or dementia, there is nothing we can do about it and there is no medication that will change it". The puzzled and angry family was
alert enough to say, "But Dr. Cath told us that you might help
by . . ." and proceeded to list an outline of what I had suggested for possible exploration. At the end of the interview, everyone left the office of this West Coast specialist feeling depressed, exhausted, angry, without vitality . If nothing truly
could be done, they and their father faced a hopelessly failing
and futile future. Furthermore, now they had little faith in the

results of any diagnostic procedures. They called back to ask
for reassurance and it was given. The years passed, the decline
was slowed if not stabilized. The patient and his family were
able to accept the realities involved and the family continued
to bring the father to see me once or twice a year.

I approach the phenomenon of depletion in the five basic
anchorages as natural processes in living long.(These include the
body, the family, the social world, economic security and (with
retirement) all too often the meaningful purposes of life. By
mid-life there is the natural coming together or convergence of
processes of depletion; these are balanced by efforts at restitution.) But I always hope every new discovery may either slow or
reverse some of these processes be they on psychological, sociological or physiological grounds. Thus, I have welcomed every
new step of every sophisticated theory involving the basic anchorages be it 1. the body and body-self, 2. the family and family
image in transition, 3. in-formation processing, 4. theories
about the meaningfullness of life, i.e. changing human capacities
for self actualization or of enhancing intimacy and sexuality.
5. new understandings of why we dream and how we sleep through
the later years for we know there is a relationship of sleep
architecture to brain integrity; 5. the significant role of nutrition related to neuro transmitter functioning or 6. any sociological factor influencing the ego-ecological system of the individual and of the physician. Thus, by utilizing the very instrument we are studying, I attempt to gather together morphological
chemical, sociological and psychological influences knowing full
well these are forces we only dimly perceive. Knowing that hu -

man life is so under the control of the most magnificent two and
a half to three pounds of integrating substance in the world, the
brain has led me to a renewed sense of awe at and respect for the
total complexity involved. Any insult to the body or body-self
be it temporary or permanent, any loss of vital supplies or input
be it sound, vision, oxygen, motility or combinations of injuries,
any organic disease with or without an array of medications, any
stress or emotional depletion, any serious relocation may have
drastic effects on mental capacities, human relatedness, the
regulation of self and the affective state in which we view our
self-object world. There is reason to believe these factors
may play a part in the response of the immune mechanisms to viral
diseases.

For the purposes of this presentation, let me start by first
summarizing some depletions in the physiological apparatus with
which and in which we live. Long ago, Shock[8] documented that
after age 35 a rate of cellular depletion of one to one and a half
percent a year is average for every organ in the body. It has
been estimated variously that we lose from 20,000 to 100,000
brain cells a day after this age; furthermore, there is a progressive slow loss of supporting glial tissue which may be equally
significant. Simultaneously, there may be an inactivating accumulation of either foreign material or endogenous toxins. While
some maintain only 10,000 brain cells are lost each day, this loss
may be related to and accelerated by toxins i.e. alcohol, nicotine,
aluminum or air pollutants. While final research figures which
would settle these rather significant ratios of loss are not in,
there is too much confirmatory reverberating evidence for us to

ignore them. Furthermore, it is significant that creativity as well as athletic prowess, for the most part, peaks in the early twenties, occasionally in the thirties . As one ages, there is a slow progressive decline in brain wave frequency and amplitude.The electroencephalogram reveals many changes in rhythm with a loss of some form of waves and lowered potentials in others. The generalized but progressive atrophy (revealed by brain scan especially by the 80's and 90's), the changed rates in cerebral blood flow all suggest changes in the basic architecture of the brain (with or without arteriosclerosis). We do know, decreased density of cells is not necessarily equivalent to efficiency of performance or the depth of meaningful experience and existence. But we also can ascertain a basic proportion of the brain must be present for clear mental functioning i.e. "counts" of the density of Alzheimers' plaques can be correlated with generalized overall performance and the progressive cerebral decline into dementia.

Thus, there is no doubt that there is a macroscopic as well as microscopic alteration in organs in terms of size, function, reserve and adaptability. All of this reflects itself in resistance to stress and/or disease as well as individual recoverability. Vulnerability may differ due to life style or characterological modes of defenses as well as intensity of change over time, i.e sudden shocks or prolonged stress, such as a series of irrecoverable losses with no chance to recover to a base line in between. In the earliest phases of depression-depletion-dementia, the patient may be intermittently aware of a loss of self and substance in declining capacities and a mournful process begins. The question of differential diagnosis may be unanswerable. Can one be depressed at a lower biological limbic level or does one need cortical and cognitive collaboration? Most believe verbal thought is not a prerequisite for depression. But one is called upon to differentiate serious regression and slowed mentation associated with depression from dementia, or sometimes from the exhausting traumatic depleting effects of a lifetime of maladjustment or disappointment, or a combination of both with serious organic illness. This differentiation may be impossible for a time and I believe there sometimes is a final common path.

I will omit from this discussion depletion in the family, the death of parents, the loss of children from the home, economic and sublimated purposes. For a complete discussion, I refer you to my previous publications.[9] Let me note another significant "late riser", the basal metabolic rate which tends to increase until about age 30. The maximum oxygen uptake and aerobic power peak between 18 and 20 and then decline. The maximum heartbeat peaks at 210 at age ten, slows to 195 at age 25, 175 at 50 and 165 at 85. Naturally enough the period of maximum adaptive capacity (in which one copes best) is the period of minimum mortality and morbidity.

It would be reasonable to assume some depletion in the capacity for physical work or in athletic capacity has to do with respiratory efficiency, cardiac stroke volume, and muscle strength. Athletes are best at short distance events early in their twenties and in endurance events between 25 and 30. However, endurance in static work in the long-lived is relatively unchanged as long as strength, small muscles and intact motor coordination remain relatively intact. Nevertheless, anytime

there is abrupt stress in older people, there will be decreased
rate of recovery from that stress.

Adaptability to cold and heat declines, as the recent fuel
shortage has so tragically demonstrated. Older people just cannot cope with the same temperature extremes as a decay of central
regulation of temperature control leads to increased mortality.
On the opposite extreme 70 percent of heatstrokes occur over the
age of 60. But you may say,as have many others, people decline,
deplete and age at different speeds. What about those who age
beautifully. Of course, there are those exceptions, whom I consider gerontocrats, who never seemingly deplete or only decline
at the very end. Furthermore, you may add,if one but enriches
the environment, one enhances overall integrity through stimulation which adds meaningfulness and years to life. To be sure, in
such a naive argument one could assert from rats in cages to human beings, one can from early to late years enlarge the size of
synapses, increase the amounts of glial material and apparently
the thickness of the cortical layer. But these are young speci-
mens and the issue for a clinician is how to deal with other than
gerontocrats with the frail, failing elders who come for help? I
ask myself, can I, in any way, alter the rate of decline, change
the quality of the later years or enhance the care of long-lived
people who have multiple disasters and diseases, depressions and
depletions to deal with and who are not gerontocrats.

There is no doubt in my mind that a universal "normal" depleting process begins in the middle of this journey through life and
takes its progressive toll in all basic anchorages. For this presentation, I have chosen to focus predominantly on the organic

because of its direct relationship between the capacity to cope
with loss and depression to resistance to disease (immunity) and
to dementia.

If we agree natural endowment (genetic) is one of the most
salient contributors to healthy endurance and intact performance
in later life, that is, one should pick one's parents from the
gerontocrats, still living long and well should never be defined
solely in genetic, chronological or functional terms. A clinical
evaluation must always include the subjective state which will in
my orientation relate predominantly to the acquired personal co-
efficients of anxiety and tolerances for depression. These will
be partially reflected in an affective stability; in a confident
sense of hope; or feelings about the short term future and the
capacity to influence it. I have learned also not to make the
error of equating maximal functional capacity with maximal adaptive capacity. Thus, while most scientific presentations attempt
to differentiate diagnoses, the major thrust of this particular
paper will be to attempt to synthesize or to bring together into
a single rubric, the strange human capacity to be depleted, depressed and demented either singly, sequentially or all at the
same time. This brings me to theory of the relationship rather
than a differential diagnosis of the foregoing depletion, depression and dementia.

With regard to the latter, most of us have observed the diagnostic lag between the onset of dementia and the time when initial medical neurological or psychiatric consultation contact is
sought. In all likelihood, dementia has an imperceptible onset
beginning from three to five years prior to the perception and

conscious recognition of any major personality or mood change.
In retrospect many families appreciated how well camouflaged and
defended they themselves were. I have only recently realized
how intact a moderately severe but pleasingly demented non-depres-
sed person may appear. In this interval of denial between the
onset of the disease and the diagnosis, an unconscious conspiracy
of concealment by the patient and the family, (and sometimes the
physician) may be due to the universal fear of insanity, the inability to think clearly and care for the self. To the human
adult,"I think therefore, I am" is a mark of his dignity. The
elder fears loss of self respect and self control, i.e. regulation of body function and of overall adaptability. He initially
may restrict his world lest "people find out" and know something
is wrong and family and social expulsion then might lead to exile
to an institution. On their part, the family may fear and resent
the burden and shame of visiting a nursing home not to mention the
considerable financial drain. Thus, there is a family need to pre-
serve the self image of an intact aged self. The family may join
in the conspiracy of denial also because of conscious and unconscious identifications with and love for the older person. They
avoid recognizing also another variant of family depletion,
the loss of a member's personhood. Historically, wives, secreta-
ries, subordinates or aides to executives or politicians have
covered up for their loved one and/or leader in more conscious
efforts to conceal his disability, lest they lose influence and
power.

    If my hypothesis, based upon more than 20 years of clinical
experience is correct, the human ego is equipped with an unappre-

ciated and unnamed psychological structure which I have called
the sensor. This "ego structure" continuously scans internal
physiological changes as well as internal psychological reserve
capacities. It measures the ideal self and self-other realized
world against accomplishments realized as well as the stresses at
hand. It is capable of intensely defending the self against all
but momentary awarenesses of the significance of changes and losses.

Some organic brain syndromes become evident because of behavioral symptoms designed to cover such sensed deficits; the defenses of confabulation and distortion. Through avoidance and
withdrawal some loss in control of skills or fine social discre-
tions may be anxiously suppressed. To the family , familiar un-
controllable mood swings may also herald a recurrence of a past
disorder and lead to the more desirable but misleading impression,
namely purely functional disease. On the other hand, uncharacteristic changes in personality, i.e. sudden irritability in a relatively calm, well adjusted president of an organization, or a well
adjusted neurologist or release of ordinarily repressed impulses
or strange behavior may be dead give-aways to familiar and significant others. Sensing changes in an elder, the spouse, children, co-workers or physician struggle with personal degrees of
gerontophobia and the universal wish to deny the evidence. Namely,
a loved person can gradually lose his personhood, his loveability
and his ability to be gratified. It is not without great pain
that most physicians come to acknowledge they are relatively or
completely impotent. They know, only too well, a diagnosis of
organic brain disease or, as I prefer to think of it, severe deple-

tion-dementia will challenge their every resource. It will possi-

bly lead, soon enough, not only to increased helplessness and

hopelessness but possibly a wish for death by everyone concerned.

What little therapeutic leverage might be present is all too fre-

quently lost sight of in the gerontophobic depressive despondency

which overtakes all participants. Although extremes may be clear

we may still not be sure what is pathological and what is normal

in the depression-depletion syndrome at any moment or age. The

peak of depression due to the characterological exhaustion-deple-

tion of the middle years (associated with suicides) is grad-

ually being matched by another peak in the early twenties. Many

more young people seem to feel terribly alienated, depleted,

bored, empty and suicidal than ever before. New research is

needed as to why these events are taking place earlier and earlier

in the life span. Some of us, based upon clinical experiences

and the teaching of Kohut[11] believe these states in supposedly

predisposed individuals (with primary disorders of self) were

results of factors in the earliest vitalizing (vs. depleting)

attaching and bonding phenomenon in the first two years of life.

These very early interactions initiate, coalesce and maintain a

basic sense of self continuity and coherency determining the to-

lerance for depression and the potential for bearing up under the

stresses and losses of later years. This balance of self-fullness

or self-emptiness is strengthened by safe unification or safe at-

taching one's self to a significant other in repeated encounters

through life. It is the quality of safe merging and of mirroring,

in repeated day to day emotionally refuelling experiences with

other significant beings (in short, healthy parenting and relating) which forms and maintains a vital enough core or primary self or a mental representational world of stored images (introjects) related to self confidence and self continuity. These factors may possibly influence the overall "jug of immunity" to help withstand the trauma and losses in each epigenetic crisis of an adult life span. Safe separation-individuation without the undue burden of parental expectations of total fusion will create enough tolerance to face the need for replacement of original objects in adolescent years and imperfection in self and idealized others. These assets may be considered the crucial precursors of the circumstances in which biochemical changes are found associated with depression. I know there are those among you who will doubt the relationship of disordered syndromes of infancy with adolescent, adult or last-trimester of life depression-depletion syndrome. I am equally sure there are those who doubt that early infantile attachments, dependencies with markedly narcissistic inclinations, often overlaid by an obsessive compulsive series of defenses may lead to vulnerability to syndromes of fragmentation, due to the problems of maintaining self coherency or holding the psychological self together, in later life. In this case, depression-depletion does take place "endogenously" or if you will, without obvious external cause or triggers. The common denominator of depression-depletion at any age is a particular vulnerability of the individual's ego, namely his inability to withstand narcissistic injury, insult or trauma.

The inward turning of larger segments of the ego apparatus which become involved in monitoring or scanning the inner workings of the body and of the self-object world, I call the "ego-

sensor". This scanning of the psycho-physiological inner world
leans heavily upon conscious memories and unconscious core introjects. It detracts available energies from outside activities
and to me explains the despair seen. This internalized structure
of earliest external experiences (nuclear versus orbital introjects in Wisdom's terms) is at the core of human individuality
and vulnerability. It seems then, the concept of depression as
endogenous or exogenous in the traditional sense represents an
artifact of conceptualization and data gathering. This is comparable to the observation that animals who have been taught to
remain immobile in the face of danger (i.e. rats immobilized after
birth in a technician's hand and then thrown into water) helplessly drown. In contrast to rats or people who have not been so
immobilized or crippled, the more fortunate of us will swim and
survive through most anything. Later core affect experiences
which represent an internal storehouse of self esteem remain operative until extreme injury to self and/or self representations
(brain cell death) threatens narcissistic balance. I will suggest
then a personal coefficient of anxiety and depression in the physician as well as the patient and family leads to states of either hopefulness or helplessness (of confident action or immobilized ambivalence) when facing a depressed, depleted-depressed
or a demented patient with various degrees of loss of brain and
self substance.

Furthermore, there is a direct relationship between anxiety,
depression, restorative sleep and brain integrity. One of the
most characteristic features of simple depression is a change in
sleep architecture and anxiety about loss of sleep refreshment.

Therefore, both patient and family suffer. Studies suggest the
least well tolerated symptoms by families is nocturnal activity
of an elder. Being awakened often leads to extreme rage, fragmentation of ego, and exhaustion of reserves and early institutionalization. Changes in sleep are almost invariably associated
with documentable biochemical changes. Alterations in sleep
architecture (or sleep profile) of the depressed patient include
a drop in sleep efficiency by 58 percent, a tendency for increased
time in falling asleep, early morning rising (reduced sleep time)
less than a total of four hours in sleep, increased wakefulness
(reduced sleep time) decreased REM latency and high REM densities.
All this suggests a great deal more mental turmoil with almost
no D time (Delta wave) sleep. A similar process of sleep fragmentation has been observed in aging and has been compared to the
sleep profiles of young psychotics. One theory goes so far as to
suppose depression at any age is a result of disturbances in in-
voluntary sleep mechanisms. Aging depressives, with physical
disease, also have less REM density, at least by 50 units. Therefore, on this basis alone it has been advised if there is high
REM density a confused, demented state should be first treated
with anti-depressants.

These various theoretical approaches have lead me to attempt
a wider synthesis of knowledge on the management of depression-
depletion-dementia which will take up my next section.

Depression Depletion Dementia - Management

The most usual method of differentiating late life confusion,
memory loss and mental distress, i.e. depression depletion and
early onset dementia, is a process of elimination. But it is my

position that these conditions can exist singly or more often as
not in various combinations of all three. Perhaps the simplest
initial approach is a thorough history and complete physical
examination as the course of the patient's life, the presence or
absence of serious neurotic or psychotic symptomatology and the
time of onset are used as critical markers. If we find a series
of earlier depressions (or other affective disturbances) or if
the timing is post-surgical etc. the idea of a pseudo or reversible dementia is immediately considered[1,2] A therapeutic trial of
restoration of familiar surroundings, antidepressants or other
symptomatic and manipulative treatments is indicated. Of some
differential value in organic dementia is excessive somatizations,
sensitivity to drugs extreme paranoid ideation or bizarreness of
symptoms. While we are also taught that hypothyroid conditions
or other systemic disturbances can simulate this state I have
not experienced this. I have learned that neuro fibrillary tangles
especially around the para-sagital sulcus, may affect the hypothalamic pituitary axis to produce a syndrome with diffuse somatic
disorganization. Our task may be still compounded by the fact
that with severe dementia there may be considerable residual cortical activity with intermittent self critical ego assessments and
exacerbation of depression. In such instances, when the depression
is adequately treated, a mild detectable residual dementia may be
found. In my opinion one of the great distortions of all time is
the idea that one of these conditions is treatable or,equally
extreme, all are untreatable, treatability depends how one defines
one's goals. I have found any one,alone, may be partially reversible and another completely so but some combinations may be to-

tally irreversible depending on <u>when</u> one comes on the scene.
However, a physician needs to carefully screen, diagnose and
decide who one is treating, how much of the whole person is
recoverable and how much the entire family can be involved. The
basis of treatability should not be on reversibility, but on
availability of ego and family resources.

It seems, in general, we have been unwilling to accept that
certain losses and diseases may coexist together each feeding on
the other and reinforcing negative therapeutic responses in all
around. To illustrate: variations in the degree of depression,
depletion and dementia are extremely important to assess. To
illustrate, a fine elderly octogenerian, developed a confusional
post operative state. The culmination of anaesthesia, hospitalization, deprivation of familiar surroundings and some inconside-
rate care-taking events within the hospital sent him into a primitive narcissistic rage. His subsequent confusion and delusional
state lasted for approximately three days despite an anti-psycho-
tic medication. During this time, his family feared his acute
confusional syndrome might become chronic and I was called in
consultation. A transfer was arranged to a nursing home where
I do visit. Within a period of two weeks under another regime
of psychotropic medications, individual and family psychotherapy,
he returned to a level of fairly calm, reasonable and better
adaptive behavior. By now a residual degree of dementia was
evident in that, he remained essentially disoriented, recent
memory was markedly impaired with immediate events selectively
failing to register and he was irritable if little things did
not go his way. When the family brought in a private duty nurse

for the evening shift, he did better. In retrospect we could
reconstruct a mild, slowly progressive, post retirement depletion-
depression and dementia had been denied for ten years and had si-
lently proceeded into a moderately severe state before his surgery.
A minor surgical procedure with general anesthesia had merely
tipped the scales beyond the adaptive capacity of his residual
cognitive and narcissistic balances. When this previously very
successful man sensed himself as helpless and hopeless, he responded with rage and was unable to function. When left alone, he
perceived his future as bleak institutionalization. With psychotherapy during the next few months, which included the family and
the nursing home staff, he gained renewed faith he had a future
with some self control, the stress of hopelessness disappeared
and there was a marked improvement in cognitive skills and memory.
Over the past year, he has remained impaired by severe arthritis
and a large inguinal hernia but his self disgust has almost disappeared and his rage at those trying to help him appropriately
selective. A pseudo dementia has turned into the residual true
depletion-dementia almost to the base line at which his surgery
began. He still requires nursing home care, but everyone is content. Thus we may see many marginally functioning individuals
stressed beyond their abilities and a pre-existing occult or
latency dementia regresses into a more chronic brain syndrome, believed to be a pseudo dementia. When such people recover, we
still find they suffer indeed from the three D's: depression,
depletion and dementia and still require great care and concern.

Conclusion

Looking into the future in the year 2020, with 20-20 vision,

it is possible to imagine we may be able to conquer the disease
of dementia. If it is truly a slow virus or an accumulation of
a toxin such as aluminum (or both) or some still unknown factor
which changes or exhausts the immune mechanisms of the human
body, victory is likely to arrive in an even shorter time. But
the power of man to seemingly stop the process of depression-
depletion seems to be less and less easy to imagine. Furthermore, our incapacity may stem from the very process of creating
humanity of human beings and the problems associated with their
disruption along with body decay and depletion. We still must
deal with the vicissitudes of many harsh realities of more long-
lived individuals in large groups all over our world. All of
this suggests a limited power to overcome depression-depletion.
Benjamin Franklin once predicted, "We may perhaps learn to de-
prive large masses of their gravity to give them absolute levity
for the sake of easy transport." (We did.) "Agriculture may
diminish its labors and double its produce." (We have done
that.) "All diseases may by sure means be prevented or cured."
(We are on our way.) Still I am forced to observe human conditions defying change. There will be in the foreseeable future
a balance between insurmountable loss and creative attempts at
restitution. Depression-Depletion-Dementia is a complex balance
with which we must struggle.

References

1. SHUR, M.   (1972) Freud Living and Dying, I.U.P., N.Y. p. 364.

2. CATH, S.H. (1966) "Beyond Depression - The Depleted State". Canadian Psychiatric Assn. J., 11:SS, S329.

3. SANDLER, J. (1959) "The Background of Safety". Proceedings of 21st Congress of the Int. Psycho-Analytical Assn.,Copenhagen.

4. BLAZER, D.G. WILLIAMS, C. (1979) "Dysphoria and Depression". NIMH study presented at the annual meeting, APA, Chicago.

5. SPITZ, R.A. (1945) "Hospitalism" The Psychoanalytic Study of the Child, I.U.P. N.Y. 1:53.

6. CATH S.H. (1965) in Geriatric Psychiatry: Grief, Loss and Emotional Disorders in the Aging Process. Cath, S.H., Berezin, M. eds., I.U.P. N.Y.

7. FREUD, S. (1961) "The Ego and the Id". Complete Works, Vol. 19, Standard Edition, Hogarth Press, p. 19.

8. SHOCK, N. (1961) in Geriatric Psychiatry: Grief, Loss and Emotional Disorders in the Aging Process. Cath, S.H., Berezin, M. eds., I.U.P. N.Y.

9. CATH, S.H. (1972) "The Institutionalization of a Parent -- a Nadir of Life." J. Geriatric Psychiatry, 5;25.

10.----(1963) "Some Dynamics of Middle and Later Years." Smith College Studies in Social Work, 33;739.

11.KOHUT, H.(1978)   "The Search for the Self , Selected Writings of Heinz Kohut."Ornstein, P. ed.,I.U.P. N.Y.

12.WELLS, C. (1979) "Pseudo-Dementia". Am J. Psychiat. 136;895.

PSYCHIATRIC SIDE-EFFECTS OF ANTIPARKINSON DRUGS

AMOS D.KORCZYN,M.D., M.Sc.* AND MELVIN D. YAHR, M.D.
Department of Neurology, Mount Sinai School of Medicine, New York, N.Y. I0029

INTRODUCTION

Psychiatric side-effects resulting from drugs used in the treatment of the elderly parkinsonian are frequent, variable and often paradoxical in type, as well as multi-factorial in origin. Their expression is determined by an interplay of the pharmacological drug action with the pathophysiologic process underlying parkinsonism, C.N.S. changes which are a consequence of aging, and the pre-morbid personality of the patient. The effects from the administration of antiparkinson medications in the elderly is influenced by their altered bioavailability, metabolism and excretion. Increased sensitivity of target and other organs may also occur particularly when concommitant diseases which are frequently encountered in this age group are present. Further, the latter frequently require treatment with medications which may interact with antiparkinson drugs, either potentiating or reducing efficacy and untoward effects. Some of the basic considerations are summarized in Tables I and 2.

Among patients manifesting symptoms of parkinsonism, idiopathic Parkinson's disease (PD) is the most commonly encountered diagnostic entity. Parkinsonism attributable to an attack of encephalitis or caused by toxic agents such as carbon monoxide or manganese is a rarity. However, parkinsonism iatrogenically induced by neuroleptic agents is common and deserves a separate discussion. Cerebral arteriosclerosis though

Supported by the Clinical Center for Research in Parkinson's and Allied Disorders NS II63I-06, The Mount Sinai School of Medicine, City University of New York, New York (Melvin D. Yahr, M.D.)
*Amos D. Korczyn, M.D., M.Sc., was the recipient of a Fellowship from the Parkinson's Disease Foundation of New York City and a Visiting Professor of Neurology at The Mount Sinai School of Medicine. His present address is Department of Physiology and Pharmacology, Tel Aviv University Medical School, Ramat Aviv, Israel.

TABLE 1

PHARMACOKINETIC FACTORS WHICH MAY INFLUENCE SIDE EFFECTS OF DRUGS IN ELDERLY PARKINSONIAN PATIENTS

1. Slow, incomplete and erratic absorption of drugs from gastro-intestinal tract.
2. Altered volume of distribution.
3. Altered drug metabolism.
4. Reduced renal clearance.
5. Altered protein binding (due to uremia, hypoalbuminemia, inter-action with other drugs, etc.).

TABLE 2

ORGAN PATHOLOGY RELATED TO SIDE EFFECTS OF ANTI-PARKINSON DRUGS IN THE ELDERLY.

Generalized neurone loss in the C.N.S.
Cardiovascular (arteriosclerosis and hypertension).
Autonomic nervous system distrubances.
Slow gastrointestinal motility.
Prostate hypertrophy.
Glaucoma.

occasionally producing symptoms resembling parkinsonism, has distinctive features and is separable from PD. It should be pointed however, that PD and cerebral arteriosclerosis not infrequently co-exist. This is of practical importance because patients with arteriosclerosis may be more vulnerable to some side effects of antiparkinson medications such as orthostatic hypotension or toxic confusional states.

It is commonly assumed that in the extrapyramidal system, an equillibrium normally exists between two neurotransmitters, acetylcholine and dopamine. In PD, degeneration of the nigro-striatal pathways leads to depletion of dopamine and thus to relative overactivity of acetylcholine. The treatment of PD is aimed at restoration of the normal balance. This can be achieved in various ways indicated in Table 3.

DRUGS USED IN THE TREATMENT OF PARKINSONISM

Prior to the 1960's the only treatment available for PD was an anti-cholinergic antimuscarinic agent. Several derivatives have been introduced, some having in addition antihistaminic properties. There is no evidence that any one of these derivatives is generally superior to others in terms

of efficacy or symptom specificity. However, individual patients

frequently prefer one agent over another, or tolerate it better.

Although there is no doubt that antimuscarinic agents are effective

to a degree, they fall far short of having a high terapeutic index. In

part this relates to their multitude of side effects. A major dis-

advantage is that patients vary widely both in control of symptoms and

vulnerability to side effects. Thus, while some patients require a dose

of I5 mg benzhexol daily, others will not tolerate even a lower dose,

manifesting side effects such as peripheral antimuscarinic blockade or

TABLE 3

DRUGS USED IN THE TREATMENT OF PARKINSON'S DISEASE

a. Drugs acting on the dopaminergic system:

    aI. Drugs which increase the availability of dopamine:
        Levodopa
        Levodopa & decarboxylase inhibitors

    a2. Direct dopamine receptor stimulants:
        Bromocriptine
        Lergotrile*
        Apomorphine*
        N-propylaporphine*

    a3. Drugs affecting dopamine release or metabolism:
        Amphetamine
        Deprenyl

b. Drugs acting on the cholinergic system**:

    Antimuscarinics

c. Drugs with unknown mechanisms of action:

    Amantadine

* not used clinically
** some of these may, in addition, block the reuptake of dopamine by nerve
   terminals

toxic delirum.

Most, and perhaps all, antimuscarinic agents have a mild euphoriant action as well as alerting responses when used in therapeutic doses.

In the elderly both the sympathetic and parasympathetic systems may be impaired[1,2]. Symptoms such as constipation, urinary retention and precipitation of glaucoma crises are more likely to follow the use of antimuscarinic agents in the elderly than in the younger age both due to the autonomic dysfunction and to the peripheral changes (e.g. prostate hypertrophy) which are common at this age. Hyperpyrexia is another risk involved in the use of high doses of these agents in the elderly, and probably reflects both peripheral blockade of sweating and central action on the temperature regulatory mechanisms.

Levodopa is the main drug presently used in parkinsonism. It serves as a precursor to dopamine. Dopamine itself does not penetrate the blood-brain barrier, and is formed in the brain only after levodopa enters the CNS. Only about 25% of an administered dose of levodopa reaches the brain, the rest being metabolized in their periphery producing dopamine and the subsequently norepinephrine. The high levels of these catecholamines are responsible for many of the side-effects of levodopa. Elderly subjects in whom sympathetic denervation is present[1], are more likely to experience these. It is possible to limit the peripheral conversion of exogenously administered dopa through the inhibition of the enzyme mediating it, dopa decarboxylase. Dopa decarboxylase inhibitors are now widely used in conjunction with levodopa; they limit the peripheral side effects which frequently have prevented the attainment of the full therapeutic potency of levodopa, and enable the use of smaller doses of levodopa, but do not otherwise modify central effects.

Other agents acting on dopaminergic receptors are the ergot alkaloids, of which only bromocriptine is presently used clinically. These are direct agonists. In some patients these new derivatives afford limited advantage over levodopa, and bromocriptine is frequently used concommitantly with levodopa, allowing smoother control of parkinsonian symptoms.

Neuroleptic agents are believed to block dopamine receptors. It is therefore clear that all neuroleptics will block the therapeutic efficacy of dopaminergic agonists, direct or indirect.

Amantadine is another important agent in the antiparkinsonian medications. Its efficacy is probably similar to that of the antimuscarinics, i.e. considerably weaker than levodopa. However, therapeutic effects are additive. The mode of action of amantadine is unclear. Increased sensitivity to amantadine side-effects occurs in old age. This may be related to renal dysfunction and impaired excretion.

Recently a new addition to the armamentarium of drugs used to treat parkinsonism has been introduced. This drug, deprenyl, belongs pharmacologically to the group of mono-amine oxidase inhibitors (MAOI). The use of MAOI in parkinsonism seems logical if one considers that the basic pathology is a deficiency in dopaminergic transmission. Indeed, various MAOI have been tried in the past but their use was forsaken because of limited efficacy and frequent side effects. Some of these, like hypotension, may be particularly common and dangerous in old age. In the last years it was established that MAO consists of two different enzymes, termed MAO-A and MAO-B. It was further shown that while the MAOI previously employed inhibited both the A and the B types of MAO, selective blockade is feasible. One agent which blocks MAO-B preferentially is deprenyl, and based on the distribution and properties of the two isoenzymes this drug was expected to be efficacious in parkinsonism while lacking most

side effects. A number of pilot studies have established that deprenyl
is in fact an effective drug [3] . These studies have further indicated that
deprenyl is helpful as an ancillary agent rather than as the sole treatment.
This is to be expected based on the pharmacological evidence that deprenyl
prevents the breakdown of dopamine, and sufficient levels of this neurotransmitter are therefore a prerequisite for deprenyl to act.

MENTAL MANIFESTATIONS IN PARKINSONISM

Patients with PD are frequently elderly and the mental side effects of
drugs which they experience must be viewed against the background of their
age and the disease. Deterioration of intellectual performance as well
as depression are common in old age; and a chronic incapacitating disease,
limiting social contact, may contribute to the affective changes. The
basic pathologic processes in PD, leading to degeneration of neural
pathways, may result in denervation supersensitivity and thus drugs may
produce excessive reactions or responses which are uncommon in normals [4] .

Mental symptoms are common in PD. Very frequently they go unreported
and undetected, mainly because patients are reluctant to volunteer the
information of hallucinations and may lack insight to intellectual
deterioration. However, careful attention and gentle suggestion reveal
most cases of hallucinations and depression. Patients will be grateful
for reassurance that they are not "getting crazy", and specific therapy or
changes of the drug regimen will be effective in a substantial proportion
of subjects.

DEMENTIA IN PARKINSON'S DISEASE
                    5
    James Parkinson in his description of the disease now bearing his name

stated that the intellect and senses were spared. With accumulated

experience, however, a strong clinical impression was formed that dementia

is more common among patients with PD than among their peers. Well-

designed and controlled studies aimed at proving this are not available,

and for good reason: Interpretation of test results in parkinsonian

patients is complicated by the motor disability, slowness of the thought

processes (bradyphrenia), frequent social isolation, mental depression

and drug effects. However, there is good evidence that short-term

memory is impaired in PD.[6] Recent data have shown that the ventricular

size is greater in PD patients as compared to controls, although this too

is at best an indirect support for the conclusion of dementia [these

studies complement previous ones demonstrating diffuse brain atrophy from
                    7   8
pneumoencephalograms and post mortem examinations].

    Upon treatment with levodopa, PD patients exhibit not only amelioration

of their physical disability but also arousal. In patients who were

severely disabled for a prolonged time this has appropriately been
                    9
described as awakening . This arousal response is probably related to

increased monoaminergic activity. In subjects with intact mentality,

this would potentiate the motor improvement in achieving a superior

beneficial response. However, when given against clouded consciousness

this alertness produced by levodopa may manifest itself as hyperactive

behavior, restlessness, agitation, aggressive behavior and hypersexuality.

In demented patients, intellectual improvement is not observed when
                    10
levodopa is administered .

    Enchancement of aminergic activity produced by levodopa is not limited

to the corpus striatum, nor is it confined to dopamine. Increased levels of norephinephrine and dopamine are observed in several brain regions in patients under chronic treatmemt. These potentiate catecholaminergic activity but may also serve as false neurotransmitters, for example in serotoninergic synapses. The implications of these alterations upon psychologic processes, if any, are still unknown. It was suggested that they may enhance the dementing process. Parkinsonian patients treated with levodopa are thought to be more demented than those seen prior to its use. It is not clear whether this is due to enhancement of the dementing process by the drug, to easier recognition of the dementia because of alertness, or a manifestation of the longer life-spans afforded by this medication.

Recently, acetylcholine has been implicated as playing a role in memory processes.[11] It is suspected that central cholinergic deficiency may under-lie at least some of the dementias. Support for this view comes from the observation that muscarinic receptor blockade within the CNS (e.g. by scopolamine) results in deficient ability to store information. Similar impairment may follow the use of antiparkinsonian agents belonging to this class of drugs. It is probable that the amnesia is reversible when treat-ment is discontinued but data to substantiate this are not available.

Several workers have demonstrated "increments" in scores obtained in a variety of psychological function tests in patients treated with levo-dopa, usually after short treatment periods. Such improvements is not necessarily due to reversal of dementia. Non-specific factors such as re-establishment of dexterity, alleviation of depressions, increased alertness and practice effects probably account for the beneficial effects (see discussion by Riklan[12]). That the improvement is more apparent than real is evident by long term studies which show a return towards baseline levels[13-16].

In some levodopa-treated patients progressive mental deterioration is observed. The time of onset of this mental dysfunction has been noted by some to begin around two years after levodopa was initiated [15].

CONFUSION AND DELIRIUM

   Confusion and delirium are toxic manifestations of several centrally acting drugs, and all antiparkinsonian agents can produce them. They typically occur following the administration of high doses, or when other precipitating factors intervene. These include high fever, CNS depressant drugs, etc. There is nothing that would characterize confusion and delirium per se resulting from one agent from those caused by another, but the occurrence of other symptoms may help (e.g. mydriatic non-responsive pupils in antimuscarinic overdose). The manifestations depend on individual factors as well as the external circumstances. For example,   confusion is likely to become more outstanding if the patient is not in his familiar surroundings.

   Delirium due to antimuscarinic drugs responds to physostigmine admini-stration. This agent inhibits cholinesterase, thus overcoming the blockade produced by the offending agents. Whether this action of physostigmine is truly specific is debatable. It has also been claimed that L-tryptophan or 5-hydroxy-tryptophan are effective in reversing levodopa induced delirium [17] but this has not been confirmed [15].

DELUSIONS

   Toxic effects of all antiparkinsonian drugs include delusions. These commonly (but not always) occur against a background of clouded conscious-ness, and very often have paranoid characteristics. They are dose depend-ent and appear at high dose levels. They should not be treated through the addition of still another drug but rather by reduction of dosage. Uncommonly complete withdrawal is required. Levodopa and ergot alkaloids induce delusions more often than other agents.

HALLUCINATIONS

Hallucinosis or hallucinations are infrequent in PD except when patients are treated. In general, these distortions of perceived stimuli are more likely to occur against a clouded consciousness such as that of a severely demented patient or in the context of toxic delirum, but they are common also in subjects with a clear sensorium.

Hallucinosis and hallucinations involving the visual system are most frequently encountered. They are most likely to occur in ambient dim light or near darkness, when interpretation of incoming optic stimuli is more difficult. The patient first recognizes these as being misconceptions, but with the progression of the symptoms finds it more and more difficult to divide the true from his imagery world. Patients frequently avoid volunteering the information that hallucinations occur.

Anticholinergics have been the major cause of hallucinations in days gone by. At the present time, the doses of these agents which are used reach toxic levels much less frequently. Levodopa produces hallucinations frequently, usually in the upper part of the terapeutic range. The prevalence of these symptoms increases progressively with prolonged use of levodopa, and at that stage they will be produced by smaller doses [15,18]. The coadministration of decarboxylase inhibitor with levodopa does not reduce or change in any other way these side effects. The pathogenesis of visual hallucinations during levodopa therapy may be related to a recently described functional defect of transmission of optic signals in PD [19].

Similar reactions occur with the other antiparkinsonian drugs. Amantadine produces hallucinations infrequently, usually when an excessive dose is used or when renal failure interferes with elimination of the drug from the body.

Ergot alkaloids tend to produce hallucinations relatively frequently. These too are usually visual, rarely auditory or olfactory [20]. It is interesting that hallucinations have not been reported when ergot deriva- tives were given for the control of endocrine disorders, and it must be recalled that these patients differ not only by their diagnoses but also by their age.

The pathogenesis of ergot-induced hallucinations has been tentatively related to a structural similarity to LSD. However, mental reactions to lergotrile and to bromocriptine are similar to those of levodopa in their characteristics as well as in the individual vulnerability to them [20], implying a common mechanism, probably related to dopamine.

It is unclear at present whether the effects of the various agents are additive, although the evidence suggests that such is the case.

AFFECTIVE RESPONSES

Depression commonly oocurs in PD. In part it is of reactive nature, as can be expected from the type and duration of the disease, the physical disability and the social isolation frequently imposed on the patients. However, there is also an element of endogenous depression. This occurs much more commonly than expected in the age group concerned. The severity of this element is of great variability among patients. The underlying mechanism is not clear but it was suggested to result from the depletion of brain amine stores.

Levodopa restores the aminergic activity towards normal, and thus would be expected to result in elimination of the depression. A detailed look at patients shows that the situation is more complex. Alleviation of the reactive element does occur as the patients realize the benefits they gain from the drug, and this in turn leads to further improvement in performance. As far as the endogenous element is concerned, however, depression does not always respond. Some patients - about 10% - react in paradoxical and unexpected deepening of the depression. These subjects may become very retarded, thus contradicting the beneficial motor effects of the drugs. Still other patients develop manic manifestations and occasionally frank manic psychosis will develop in response to levodopa. Patients with previous history of affective disorders, either in themselves or in first degree relatives are particularly susceptible [21].

Antimuscarinic agents have weak mood-elevating effects. Amantadine does not seem to cause affective changes.

In a depressed patient with PD, changes of environmental conditions must be attempted, such as socialization. These will probably ameliorate the reactive element. For the endogenous element which does not respond to levodopa, tricyclic antidepressants can be added and occasionally are quite helpful. It should be recorded that these agents also have intrinsic antimuscarinic actions which may improve parkinsonism but also can cause side effects alone or by potentiating the actions of anti-cholinergic drugs administered concurrently.

Electroconvulsive treatment has no place in the care of the depressed patient with PD. MAOI are also contraindicated, particularly in patients on levodopa therapy, because of imminent interactions. Whether selective inhibitors, like deprenyl, affect mood is still unknown. In patients with cyclic affective disorder, the use of lithium can be initiated or continued without apparent interaction with the antiparkinsonian medication.

CONCLUSION

From the foregoing it is evident that mental side-effects occurring in parkinsonian patients receiving therapeutic agents for their disease are frequent and diverse in nature. The effects observed are not determined solely by the pharmacological agents. Multiple aspects of parkinsonism intervene and account for reactions which may not occur when such medications are administered to non-parkinsonians. Thus it is necessary to view the drug-effect reactions within the context of the patient, his age, the premorbid personality and the organic and functional changes which have occurred as a consequence of the parkinsonian state as well as co-existing disorders. These factors may fluctuate in degree and their interaction therefore results in mental expressions which vary not only from patient to patient, but also at various times in each individual subject.

REFERENCES

1. Korczyn, A.D., Laor, N., and Nemet, P. (1976) Arch. Ophthalmol. 94, 1905-1906.
2. Korczyn, A.D. and Laor, N. (1976) Isr. J. Med. Sci. 12, 1525.
3. Birkmayer, W., Riederer, P., and Youdim, M.B.H. (1975) J. Neurol. Transm. 36, 303.
4. Korczyn, A.D. (1972) Neuropharmacol. 11, 601.
5. Parkinson, J. (1817) An Essay on the Shaking Palsy. Sherwood, Neely and Jones, London.
6. Bowen, F.P. (1976) in The Basal Ganglia, Yahr, M.D. ed., Raven Press, New York, pp 169-177.
7. Selby, G. (1968) J. Neurol. Sci. 6, 517-559.
8. Forno, L.S. and Alvord, E.C. (1971) in Recent Advances in Parkinson's Disease, McDowell, F.H. and Markham, C.H., ed., pp 119-162.
9. Sacks, O.W. (1973) Awakenings, Duckworth, London, pp 1-255.
10. Mones, R.J., Elizan, T.S. and Siegel, G.S. (1970) N.Y. St. J. Med. 70, 2309-2318.
11. Drachman, D.A. and Leavitt, J. (1974) Arch. Neurol. 30, 113-121.
12. Riklan, M. (1973) L-Dopa and Parkinsonism, a Psychological Assessment. Charles C. Thomas, Springfield, pp 1-402.
13. Botez, M.I. and Barbeau, A. (1973) Lancet, 2, 1028-1029.
14. Loranger, A.W., Goodell, H. and McDowell, F.H. (1973) Am. J. Psychiat. 130, 1386-1389.
15. Sweet, R.D., McDowell, F.H., Geigenson, J.S., Loranger, A.W. and Goodell, H. (1976) Neurol. (Minneap.) 26, 305-310.

16.Bowen, F.P., Burns, M.M. and Yahr, M.D. (1976) in Advance in
   Parkinsonism, Birkmayer, W. and Hornykiewitz, O. ed., Roche, Basle,
   pp 488-491.
17.Birkmayer, N. and Neumayer, E. (1972) Nervenarzt, 43, 76-78.
18.Moskovitz, C., Moses, H. and Klawans, H.L. (1978) Am. J. Psychiat.
   135, 669.
19.Bodis-Wollner, I. and Yahr, M.D. (1979) Brain, 101, 661-671.
20.Lieberman, A., Estey, E., Kupersmith, M., Gopinathan, G. and Goldstein,
   M. (1978) J. Amer. Med. Assoc. 238, 2380-2382.
21.Mendlewitz, J., Yahr, F. and Yahr, M.D. (1976) in Advances in
   Parkinsonism, Birkmayer, W. and Hornykiewitz, O. ed. Roche, Basle, pp
   103-107.

III
Newer Groups of Drugs

Published 1979 by Elsevier North Holland, Inc.
Nandy, Ed. Geriatric Psychopharmacology

ERGOT DERIVATIVES AND THE CENTRAL NERVOUS SYSTEM: EFFECTS OF CO-DERGOCRINE
MESYLATE (HYDERGINE®) ON CEREBRAL SYNAPTIC TRANSMISSION

D.M. LOEW, J.M. VIGOURET AND A.L. JATON
Preclinical Research, Pharmaceutical Division, Sandoz Ltd., CH-4002, Basel
Switzerland

SUMMARY

A review of the *in vitro* effects of Co-dergocrine mesylate (dihydroergotoxine
mesylate, Hydergine®) shows that the drug can compete with radioligands for the
occupation of specific binding sites of NA, DA and 5-HT in the brain. In
addition, Hydergine counteracts the elevation of cyclic AMP content of brain
tissue induced by NA or DA. *In vivo*, an acceleration of NA turnover, and a
slowing of DA and 5-HT brain turnover suggest NA antagonist, DA agonist and 5-
HT agonist effects. In functional tests evidence is available for agonist
effects of Hydergine at central DA and 5-HT receptors. Investigations after
repeated administration indicate that some effects of Hydergine on cognitive
behaviour and on neurobiochemical regulation become more pronounced which is
proposed to be due to an accumulation in brain tissue or an enhanced sensitivity
of central receptor sites.

INTRODUCTION

A recent review of the effects of ergot derivatives on the central nervous
system indicates rapid progress in research on the effects of these compounds
on synaptic transmission in recent years[1]. The example of bromocriptine (Par-
lodel®) shows how the observation by K. FUXE that bromocriptine exerts a dopamine (DA) agonist effect on the nigrostriatal system in rats[2], has led to its
use in the treatment of parkinsonism[3]. LSD-25, the diethylamide derivative of
lysergic acid, has also been the subject of numerous studies on synaptic transmission. Earlier, LSD-25 was proposed to be a selective central serotonin (5-HT)
agonist[4]. We now assume that the effect of this compound on synaptic transmission is more complex since it appears to act partly as a 5-HT, partly as a
DA agonist[5,6]. Practically all that was known of the dihydrogenated peptide
alkaloids of ergot was their peripheral noradrenaline (NA) antagonist properties
described in the now classical papers of ROTHLIN[7]. Only in 1975, MARKSTEIN and

WAGNER[8] demonstrated that Hydergine®,* a typical representative of this group
of ergot alkaloids exerted effects on cerebral synaptic transmission. In
addition, investigations under conditions of impaired brain metabolism indicated
that Hydergine, by activating brain metabolism, may protect the brain from some
of the consequences of temporary ischemia or hypoxia[9,10].

The pharmacological effects of Hydergine in various functional tests, such as
the sleep-wakefulness cycle and the behaviour of intact rats and of rats with
localised cerebral lesions, the ponto-geniculo-occipital (PGO) waves, its emetic
effects in dogs and its inhibition of the antinociceptive activity of morphine
in rabbits, can be explained in terms of various changes in central synaptic
transmission[1,11,12,13]. As compared to bromocriptine, whose functional effects
can be best explained on the basis of a dopamine agonist action[14], it is not yet
clear whether all of the functional effects of Hydergine can be traced back to
an action at known synaptic receptor sites. Comparative studies with four ergot
derivatives[15,16] suggest that a 5-HT agonist action is typical of Hydergine
whereas its DA agonist effects appear less important. In addition, none of the
effects of Hydergine in these functional tests appears to reflect the NA antagonist activity found by biochemical methods[8,17]. The beneficial effects of Hydergine in the treatment of symptoms of cerebrovascular insufficiency and senile
dementia[18,19] justifies a thorough analysis of its effect on the cerebral monoaminergic systems. In fact the numerous results obtained in animals and human
subjects suggest that in senile and other cerebral disorders occurring in old
age, there are age-related changes in central neurotransmission[20].

The effect of Hydergine on central synaptic transmission may be investigated
in two different ways - *in vitro* and *in vivo*. *In vitro* studies relate to the
properties involved in physico-chemical binding to specific receptor sites in
the brain and in modifying the activity of adenylate cyclase - one of the links
in the chain of neuronal transmission. *In vivo* studies make use of biochemical
and functional techniques, which reveal pharmacodynamic effects in the whole
animal. An analysis of the results obtained by these two types of study offers
a means of seeking correlations between the pharmacodynamic and therapeutic properties of Hydergine.

---

*Co-dergocrine mesylate (BAN) or Hydergine® is comprised of equal parts of the
mesylates of dihydroergocornine, dihydroergocristine and dihydroergokryptine,
the latter in the form of its α- and β-isomers in the proportion of 2 to 1.

IN VITRO STUDIES

The effects exerted by Hydergine *in vitro* have been investigated by two different types of experiments. A study of the ability of Hydergine to displace known radioactive ligands from their specific binding sites in homogenates of cerebral structure may provide information on the similarity between the physico-chemical properties of Hydergine and those of standard substances, and on the affinity of Hydergine for specific cerebral tissues. Secondly, we have studied how Hydergine interacts with agents stimulating adenylate cyclase activity. This experiment provides information on the effect of Hydergine on synaptic transmission. Adenylate cyclase, an enzyme present on the surface of the cell membrane, converts adenosine triphosphate (ATP) to cyclic adenosine monophosphate (cAMP) which is believed to be the second messenger responsible for the hormonal response. It should be noted, however, that it is not certain whether this is the case for all neurons.

Noradrenaline receptors

Previous studies have shown that ^{3}H-dihydroergokryptine binds readily and specifically to rabbit uterine membranes. These sites are reported to possess characteristics similar to those of alpha-adrenoceptors[21]. The affinity of Hydergine for alpha-adrenoceptors was then estimated indirectly by measuring the competition between ^{3}H-dihydroergokryptine and Hydergine for the binding sites on rat cortical membranes[22]. Hydergine was found to have a high affinity for the ^{3}H-dihydroergokryptine receptor sites (K_i : 30nM). This effect was comparable to that of alpha-adrenoceptor antagonists such as phentolamine (K_i : 75 nM) or WB-4101 (K_i : 23 nM). Hydergine does not owe this effect to its chemical similarity with dihydroergokryptine, since Hydergine still more effectively antagonises the binding of ^{3}H-WB-4101, (2', 6'-dimethoxyphenoxyethylaminomethyl benzidoxane) to the receptor sites (Table I). BUERKI et al.[16] have confirmed that

TABLE I

INHIBITION OF BINDING TO RAT BRAIN CORTICAL MEMBRANES (22)

Compounds	^{3}H-WB-4101 K_i (nM)	^{3}H-dihydroergokryptine K_i (nM)
WB-4101	0.75	23
Dihydroergokryptine	3.8	15
Phentolamine	9.5	75
Haloperidol	48	-
Hydergine	6.7	30
Bromocriptine	9.5	470

Hydergine is effective in inhibiting ^{3}H-dihydroergokryptine binding and have demonstrated that it only weakly inhibits ^{3}H-alprenolol which binds to β-adrenergic receptors.

The first clues that Hydergine had an effect on cortical adenylate cyclase which is sensitive to NA came from experiments in rats which had been treated for two years at a daily oral dosage of 6.2 mg/kg (males) and 3.1 mg/kg (females). The cAMP content of the cerebral cortex and cerebellum was found to be significantly reduced[23]. *In vitro* studies on slices of rat cortex show that Hydergine inhibits the increase in cAMP level induced by NA (Fig.1). This effect of NA is

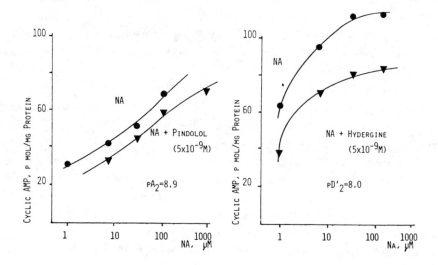

Fig.1. Antagonism by pindolol and Hydergine of the elevation of cyclic AMP content of rat cerebral cortex slices[17].

inhibited competitively by compounds known to be selective inhibitors of α- or β-adrenoceptors, while the inhibition by Hydergine is non-competitive since it cannot be surmounted even by high concentrations of NA[8,17]. Furthermore, since the rise in cAMP level brought about by isoproterenol or adenosine is not reversed by Hydergine, its action on the NA receptors in this model may be regarded as selective; the affinity of Hydergine for the NA receptor is approximately 10.000 times greater than its affinity for the other two types of receptor sites (Table II). Hence this experiment demonstrates that Hydergine may antagonise NA at NA receptors, but that this effect differs from that of α- and β-adrenoceptor blocking agents.

TABLE II

CYCLIC AMP LEVELS (A) AND RECEPTOR AFFINITIES (B) IN SLICES OF RAT CEREBRAL
CORTEX[17].

A. Cyclic AMP levels
   (pmol/mg protein)

Agonist	Concentration (μM)	Agonist	Agonist + Hydergine (1 μM)
Isoproterenol	0	10.9 ± 1.3	–
	0.5	24.1 ± 0.7	20.8 ± 2.6
Noradrenaline	0	8.5 ± 1.0	–
	0.5	47.8 ± 4.1	21.9 ± 1.2
Adenosine	0	17.3 ± 2.0	–
	25	93.4 ± 8.7	84.4 ± 4.0

B. Affinity for the receptors
   (pA_2 or $pD_2'*$)

Antagonist	Agonist		
	Noradrenaline	Isoproterenol	Adenosine
Phentolamine	7.9	< 4	–
Pindolol	8.9	9.0	–
Hydergine*	8.0	< 4	< 4

Dopamine receptors

The affinity of Hydergine for the presynaptic DA receptors was estimated indirectly by measuring tyrosine hydroxylase activity in the synaptosomes of the
rat striatum[22,24]. Hydergine weakly supressed tyrosine hydroxylase activity.
This effect is characteristic of DA agonists such as apomorphine and bromo-
crtiptine. Furthermore, Hydergine also counteracts the effects of apomorphine
in this experiment. It would appear, therefore, that Hydergine possesses moderate activity at presynaptic DA receptors and may act both as an agonist and
as an antagonist.

The affinity of Hydergine for brain DA receptors has been assessed by measuring the competition between ^{3}H-DA and Hydergine for specific binding sites in cell membranes of bovine striatum and between Hydergine and ^{3}H-haloperidol in the rat striatum[22]. Like apomorphine, Hydergine and bromocriptine displace DA and haloperidol from their specific binding sites in the caudate nucleus[22,25]. BUERKI[25] has shown that in their capacity to inhibit the binding of haloperidol in the rat caudate nucleus, Hydergine and bromocriptine display a much greater affinity than apomorphine and DA (Table III).

TABLE III

INHIBITION OF BINDING OF ^{3}H-HALOPERIDOL TO THE MEMBRANES OF THE RAT CAUDATE NUCLEUS[25].

Compounds	IC_{50} (nM)
Haloperidol	0.5
Apomorphine	40
Dopamine	2200
Noradrenaline	> 10000
Serotonin	> 10000
Hydergine	3
Bromocriptine	3

Studies of the effects of Hydergine on the affinity of DA-sensitive adenylate cyclase have furnished contradictory results. From the *in vitro* studies of SPANO and TRABUCCHI[26], it emerges that Hydergine inhibits the increase in cAMP induced by DA and apomorphine (Fig.2.), but that it is less effective than bromocriptine in this respect (Table IV). On the other hand, at higher concentrations, Hydergine facilitates the formation of cAMP *in vitro* in the isolated rabbit retina[27,28]. In addition, PORTALEONE[29] reported that the administration of 3 mg/kg Hydergine i.p. is a moderate stimulus to the formation of cAMP in the rat striatum. It should be added that unlike the neuroleptic agents, notably haloperidol, Hydergine reduces DA inhibition of spontaenous neuronal activity induced in the snail Helix aspersa[30].

There is still some debate on whether ergot derivatives such as Hydergine or bromocriptine, at the DA receptor level, behave as agonists or antagonists. Recently, Kebabian and Calne[31] have tried to resolve the issue by proposing two types of DA receptors. Ergot derivatives would act as antagonists at the D-1 receptor which depends on adenylate cyclase. At the D-2 receptor ergot derivatives would have agonist actions but the D-2 receptor is independent of adenylate cyclase activation.

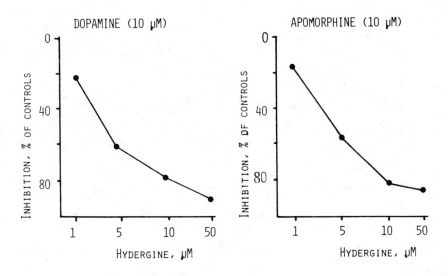

Fig. 2. Antagonism of dopamine induced cyclic AMP elevation in the rat striatum[26].

TABLE IV

ANTAGONISM OF THE DOPAMINE INDUCED INCREASE IN CYCLIC AMP IN THE RAT STRIATUM[26]

Compounds	IC_{50} (μM)
Hydergine	3.3
Bromocriptine	0.75
Ergotamine	0.7
Dihydroergotamine	0.5

Serotonin receptors

It is not surprising that ergot derivatives should be capable of displacing 5-HT from its binding sites in the brain. Some years ago BENNETT and SNYDER[32] demonstrated that compounds with a structure resembling that of LSD-25 displaced 5-HT. The investigations of CLOSSE and HAUSER[33] show that 5-HT possesses an affinity for the binding sites of ^{3}H-dihydroergotamine greater than NA (Fig.3).

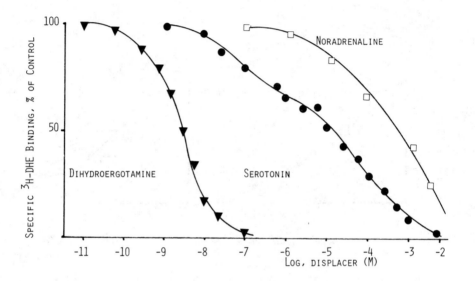

Fig. 3. Inhibtion of binding of ^{3}H-dihydroergotamine to rat brain membranes[33].

The 5-HT displacement curve displays an irregular shape which is believed to reflect the sum of two displacement curves. This may indicate that ^{3}H-dihydroergotamine binds to two different specific possibly 5-HT binding sites. As seen in Table V, Hydergine displaces dihydroergotamine and 5-HT in concentrations of about 10 nM and 200 nM, respectively.

IN VIVO STUDIES

The *in vivo* studies comprise neurobiochemical investigation of the metabolism of biogenic and behavioural studies in which the effects of Hydergine have been compared with those of DA and 5-HT agonists and precursors.

TABLE V

INHIBITION OF BINDING OF ^{3}H-DIHYDROERGOTAMINE AND ^{3}H-SEROTONIN TO RAT BRAIN
MEMBRANES[33] and unpublished results of CLOSSE and HAUSER.

Drug	IC_{50} (nM)	
	[3]H- dihydroergotamine	^{3}H-serotonin
Dihydroergotamine	4	6
Hydergine	12	200
Bromocriptine	135	255

Neurobiochemical investigations

Hydergine alters the levels of metabolites of the biogenic amines in the rat
brain (Fig.4). The breakdown of NA is accelerated, this accounting for a higher
level of 4-hydroxy-3-methoxy-phenyl-ethylene sulphate (MOPEG.SO$_4$) in the rat
brain stem. Furthermore, the concentration of 3,4-dihydroxy-phenyl acetic acid
(DOPAC), the principal metabolite of DA, in the striatum is depressed, as is
the concentration of 5-hydroxy-indole-acetic acid (5-HIAA) in the cerebral cortex[15,16].

Changes in the concentrations of the metabolites of endogenous amines are
attributed to postsynaptic effects of exogenous coumpounds. The increase in
MOPEG is thought to be related to an NA antagonist effect of Hydergine at the
postsynaptic receptors. As a result a negative feedback system is inhibited,
this stimulating the synthesis and breakdown of NA. Nevertheless, it is also
possible that Hydergine might liberate NA from the presynaptic terminals. The
reduction in DOPAC and 5-HIAA levels is regarded as an indication that Hydergine exercices postsynaptic agonist effects on the DA and 5-HT receptors. Such
an agonist effect would reinforce the negative feedback mechanism thereby reducing the synthesis and breakdown of DA and 5-HT. It should be added that Hydergine does not affect the concentrations of DA and 5-HT, while it antagonises
biochemical effects of morphine, haloperidol and clozapine[12].

Behavioural studies: Dopamine agonist effects

A large number of experimental models are available for the study of the dopaminergic systems. In dogs Hydergine has a particularly pronounced emetic action (ED 50: 5.7 µg/kg i.v.). According to PAPP et al.[34] and SHARE et al.[35]
the mechanism involved in this effect closely resembles that responsible for

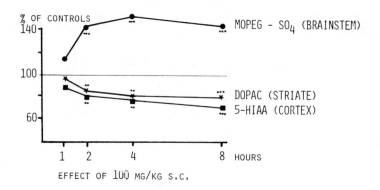

EFFECT OF 100 MG/KG S.C.

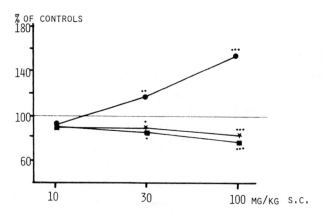

Fig.4. Effects of Hydergine on metabolites of biogenic amines in the rat brain[16].

the effect of the DA agonist apomorphine. Like apomorphine, Hydergine induces contralateral turning behaviour in rats with unilateral lesions of the nigro-striatal pathways induced by administering 6-hydroxy-dopamine into the substantia nigra[15]. It will be seen from Fig 5 that the effect of Hydergine does not make its onset for a period of two hours and that the active dose is appreciably greater that that of bromocriptine. Nevertheless, the active doses of Hydergine in the Ungerstedt model are similar to those which reduce the DOPAC levels. In doses up to 100 mg/kg s.c., Hydergine does not induce apomorphine like stereo-typed behaviour in the rat. Moreover, in doses up to 30 mg/kg s.c., Hydergine does not inhibit the akinesia induced by reserpine in the mouse[15]. Nevertheless, similar to apomorphine or bromocriptine, Hydergine inhibits α-rigidity at an ID_{50} of 0.85 mg/kg i.v.[36], in rats treated with 10 mg/kg i.v. reserpine.

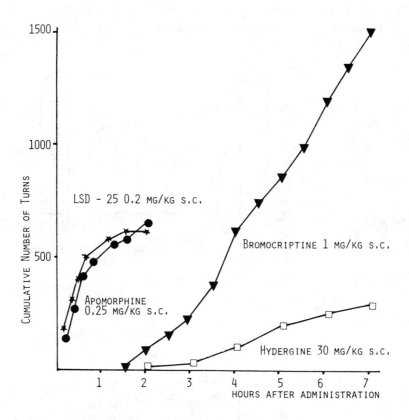

Fig.5. Induction of contralateral turning behaviour in rats with unilateral lesions of the nigrostriatal pathways.

The intravenous administration of various DA agonists such as apomorphine, bromocriptine and d-amphetamine reduces the antinociceptive effect of morphine in rabbits[11,15]. A comparable reduction is observed after administration of Hydergine (2.5 to 10 mg/kg i.v.). Hydergine differs from these DA agonists in that its effect is manifest at doses which do not give rise to increase motor activity. Furthermore, intraventricular administration of the DA-antagonist pimozide shows that the effect due to Hydergine involves dopaminergic pontomedullary structures in the vicinity of the 4th ventricle (Fig.6). Several authors have demonstrated that Hydergine is able to attenuate the injurious effects of acute cerebral ischemia or general hypoxia in animals[10,37-40]. This protective effect of Hydergine could be related to a DA agonist effect since L-DOPA or an increase in the cerebral DA level reduces the injurious effect of hypoxia[41,42]. Moreover,

184

in common with L-DOPA, apomorphine and bromocriptine, Hydergine partly reverses the behavioural changes induced in rats by hypoxia[43,44].

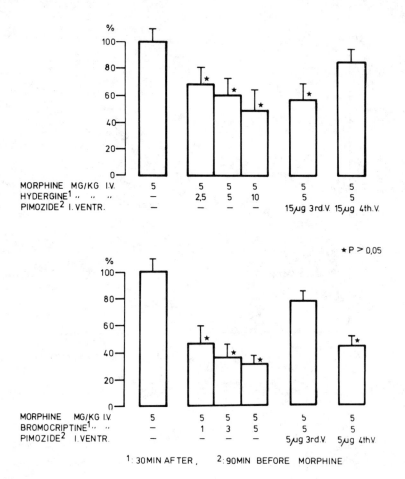

Fig.6. Antagonism of the antinociceptive effects of morphine in the rabbit[15].

Behavioural studies: Serotonin agonist effects

Apart from reduction in 5-HT metabolism, certain other effects of Hydergine resemble those induced by 5-hydroxytryptophan (5-HTP) and this is considered to be evidence of a 5-HT agonist effect. Changes in the sleep-wakefulness cycle in the rat induced by low doses of Hydergine are similar to those observed after administration of 5-HTP (Fig.7). Unlike stimulants of the d-amphetamine type, Hydergine and 5-HTP do not give rise to increase motor activity. Moreover, they have only a limited capacity to prolong wakefulness and reduce non-REM sleep.

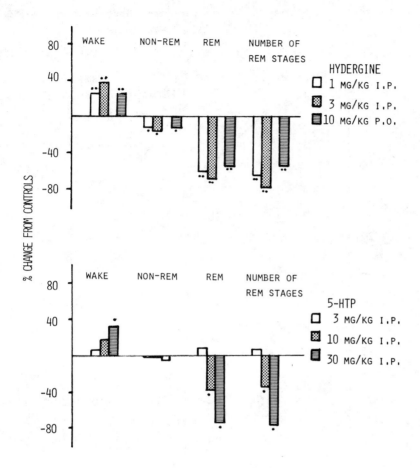

Fig.7. Effects of Hydergine and 5-HTP on the sleep-wakefulness cycle of the rat.[12]

The reduction in the duration of REM sleep is mainly due to a reduction in the number of phases[12,13].

The administration of reserpine to cats induces high voltage electrical potentials in the pons (P), lateral geniculate body (G) and occipital cortex (O), which are called PGO waves. They result from depletion of monoamines, especially 5-HT from storage granules. Serotonin depletion probably releases the activity of a pace-maker in the pons which generates rhythmic discharges at a frequency of 30-50/minute. Administered in cumulative doses, Hydergine reduces the number of PGO waves similarly to 5-HTP (Fig.8). At the same time the two substances reverse the effect of reserpine on cortical EEG activity[11]. Pretreat-

186

ment with methiothepin, a central serotonin antagonist, displaces the dose-effect
curve of the two compounds to the right whereas phenoxybenzamine or pimozide did

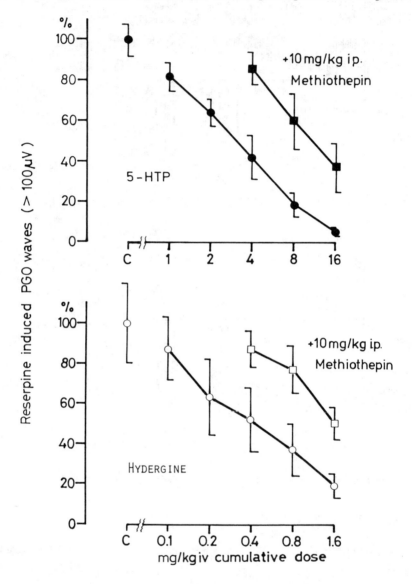

Fig.8. Displacement of the dose-effect curves of 5-HTP and Hydergine by prior
administration of methiothepin. PGO waves in tne reserpinised cat[45].

not displace the dose-response curves[45]. It has therefore been postulated that

Hydergine has either a 5-HT agonist effect on the cells of the raphe nuclei, or imitates the effects of 5-HT on the thalamic nuclei, which are rich in serotoninergic terminals. AGHAJANIAN demonstrated that LSD-25 acts as these two sites[46].

Behavioural studies: Effects on goal-directed behaviour

Recently, we have investigated the effects of repeated administration of Hydergine on rats which were trained to receive food by working in a Lashley maze[36,47]. The drug was given before each of 4 consecutive trials. Control rats, trained under identical conditions learned to perform the task as indicated by a reduction in starting time (ST), running time (RT) and number of errors (NE) over the 4 day period. The daily administration of 3 mg/kg s.c. of Hydergine, 4 hours before trial, resulted in a further reduction of ST, RT and NE. As compared to control animals these effects became more accentuated as the number of trials and administration increased (Fig.9).

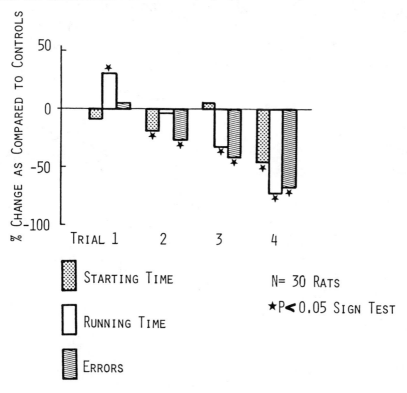

Fig.9. Effects of 3 mg/kg s.c. of Hydergine on maze learning in the rat[36].

When Hydergine was given 2 hours before trial, NE was still reduced, but ST and RT were enhanced (Fig.10).

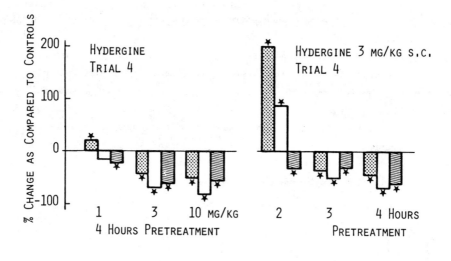

Fig.10. Effects of various doses and pretreatment times on maze learning. For explanation of symbols see fig.9.

These results show that the effects on learning a goal directed behaviour are not directly correlated to motor inhibition or motor excitation. In the maze learning experiment it appears that Hydergine enhances cognitive performance i.e. the ability of rats to discriminate environmental stimuli, and that this effect is independent of changes in motor performance.

Comparison of *in vitro* and *in vivo* studies

   In vitro studies have shown that at low concentrations of around 10^{-8} M, Hydergine displaces radioactive ligands from their central binding sites and inhibits the increase in cyclic AMP induced by catecholamines. It follows from these investigations that the central receptor sites for Hydergine may be those also occupied by NA, DA and 5-HT.

   Nevertheless, it is surprising to note that *in vivo* Hydergine has to be administered in relatively high doses. Depending upon the test and the animal em-

ployed, these doses vary from 0.2 mg/kg i.v. to 30 and 100 mg/kg i.p. This observation is all the more surprising as the Hydergine dosage recommended for human subjects amounts to only a few milligrams per day. However, it should be
borne in mind that in the treatment of senile behavioural disorders, the beneficial effects of Hydergine do not become apparent until the patient has been
treated for several weeks.

It is necessary to stress here, that the pharmacodynamic properties of a compound employed therapeutically are generally investigated in acute experiments,
i.e. after administration of a single dose to a laboratory animal. Such a procedure is justifiable when the compound in question has an instant therapeutic
effect in human subjects after administration of a single dose. Since this is
not the case for Hydergine, we have investigated its spectrum of pharmacological activities after repeated administration. Besides the studies in rats on the
effects of repeated administration of Hydergine on maze learning[36,47] and a two
years oral study summarized recently by RICHARDSON[48], two other investigations
have demonstrated that the effects of Hydergine emerge more clearly after repeated administration.

MARKSTEIN and WAGNER[17] gave Hydergine to rats at a daily oral dosage of 3 mg/
kg for 6 weeks. They sacrificed the animal 1, 3 and 6 weeks after the start of
treatment in order to investigate the effect exerted by Hydergine on the increase in cAMP level induced *in vitro* by NA in slices of cortex (Fig.11). The controls showed a well defined increase in sensitivity to NA. This enhancement of
sensitivity was absent in the animal undergoing prolonged treatment with Hydergine. MARKSTEIN and WAGNER assume that Hydergine accumulates in the rat brain
when given for a number of weeks. The cumulative concentration was calculated to
be 10^{-8}M, precisely the same concentration which had previously been found to be
effective in *in vitro* studies of Hydergine (see Fig.1).

In a second experiment (Fig.12) we administered the same oral dose of Hydergine twice, with an interval of 24 hours, to rats with unilateral degeneration
of the nigrostriatal pathways. As we have already noted (see Fig.5), the first
dose of Hydergine induced weak turning behaviour contralateral to the lesion.
After the second dose on the following day, the turning behaviour, as measured
by the total number of turning movements, was considerably increased, while the
latency period noted on the first day was markedly shortened. An increase in
response of this nature was only observed when the initial dose was capable of
inducing at least a liminal effect. These results suggest that the first dose of
Hydergine enhances the sensitivity of the central sites responsible for these
effects. Changes in the sensitivity of cerebral dopaminergic sites have been
described after denervation brought about by chemical lesions[50] and after

190

administration of neuroleptics[51,52]; and indeed such changes may be induced by administration of a single dose of a DA agonist, e.g. apomorphine[53]. These results confirm the need to investigate the effects of Hydergine during long-term administration, since it appears that the effects of the compound are then enhanced. This phenomenon may be attributed to accumulation of Hydergine or to sensititation of its central sites of action.

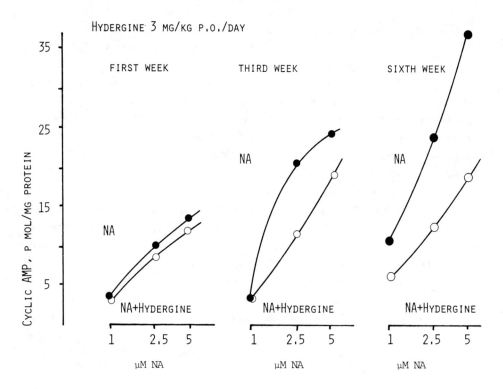

Fig.11. Antagonism by Hydergine on the elevation of cyclic AMP content of rat cerebral cortex slices[17]. o--o Hydergine 3 mg/kg/day p.o. ●--● Placebo.

ACKNOWLEDGEMENT

This manuscript has been published in an earlier version in Interdiscipl. Topics Geront. 15, 85-103, 1979. The authors thank Dr. Fritz Karger for his permission to republish parts of this text.

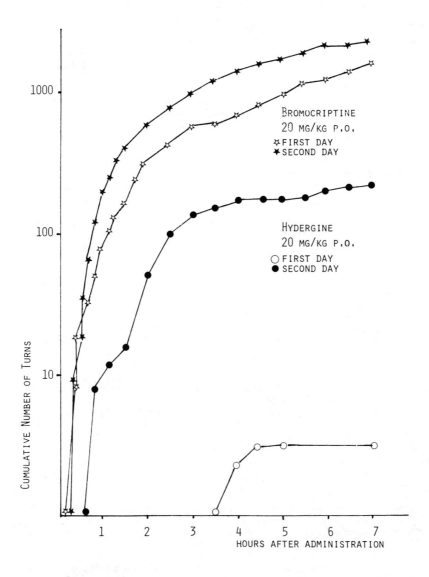

Fig.12. Induction of contralateral turning behaviour in rats with unilateral lesions of the nigrostriatal pathways. Administration of Hydergine and Bromo-criptine on two consecutive days[49].

REFERENCES

1. Loew, D.M., van Deusen, E.B. and Meier-Ruge. W. (1978) in Ergot Alkaloids and Related Compounds, Berde, B. and Schild, H.O., ed., Handbuch der experimentellen Pharmakologie 49, 421-532.

2. Corrodi, H., Fuxe, K., Hökfelt, T., Lidbrink, P. and Ungerstedt, U. (1973) J. Pharm. Pharmac. 25, 409-412.
3. Calne, D.B. (1976) The New England J. Med. 295, 1433-1434.
4. Freedman, D.X. (1961) J. Pharmacol. exp. Therap. 134, 160-166.
5. Pieri, L., Pieri, M.and Haefely, W. (1974) Nature 252, 586-588.
6. Von Hungen, K., Roberts, D. and Hill, D.F. (1974) Nature, 252, 588-589.
7. Rothlin, E. (1946/47) Bull. Schweiz. Akad. med. Wiss. 2, 249-272.
8. Markstein, R. and Wagner, H. (1975) FEBS Letters, 55, 275-277.
9. Emmenegger, H., Meier-Ruge, W. (1968) Pharmacology, 1, 65-78.
10. Meier-Ruge, W., Enz, A., Gygax, P., Hunziker, O., Iwangoff, P. (1975) in Genesis and Treatment of Psychological Disorders in the Elderly, Gershon, S., Raskin, A. ed. Raven Press, New York, pp.55-126.
11. Depoortere, H., Loew, D.M. and Vigouret, J.M. (1975) Triangle, 14, 73-79
12. Loew, D.M., Depoortere, H. and Bürki, H.R. (1976) Arneim.- Forsch. (Drug Res.), 26, 1080-1083.
13. Loew, D.M., Jaton, A.L. and Vigouret, J.M. (1976) Postgrad. Med. J., 52, Suppl. 1. 40-46.
14. Clark, B., Flückiger, E., Loew, D.M., Vigouret, J.M. (1978) Triangle, 17, 21-31.
15. Vigouret, J.M., Bürki, H.R., Jaton, A.L., Züger, P.E. and Loew, D.M. (1978) Pharmacology, 16, Suppl. 1, 156-173.
16. Bürki, H.R., Asper, H., Ruch, W. and Züger, P.E. (1978) Psychopharmacology, 57, 227-237.
17. Markstein, R. and Wagner, H. (1978) Gerontology, (Basel), 24, Suppl. 1, 94-105.
18. Venn, R.D. (1978) in Ergot Alkaloids and Related Compounds, Berde, B., Schild, H.O. ed., Handbuch der experimentellen Pharmakologie,49, 533-566.
19. Fanchamps, A. (1980) Controlled studies with dihydroergotoxine in senile cerebral insufficiency. This voulume.
20. Samorajski,T. (1977) Amer. Geriat. Soc., 25, 337-348.
21. Williams, L.T. and Lefkowitz, R.J. (1976) Science, 192, 791-793.
22. Goldstein, M., Lew, J.Y., Hata, F. and Liebermann, A. (1978) Gerontology (Basel), 24, Suppl.1, 76-85.
23. Enz, A., Iwangoff, P., Markstein, R. and Wagner, H. (1975) Triangle, 14, 90-92.
24. Lew, J.Y., Ohashi, T. and Goldstein, M. (1976) Pharmacologist, 18, Abstract 113, 134.
25. Bürki, H.R. (1978) Unpublished results.
26. Spano, P.F. and Trabucchi, M. (1978) Gerontology (Basel), 24, Suppl.1, 106-114.
27. Schorderet, M. (1977) Unpublished results.
28. Schorderet, M. (1978) Gerontology (Basel), 24, Suppl.1, 86-93.
29. Portaleone, P. (1978) Pharmacology, 16, Suppl. 1, 207-209.
30. Struyker-Boudier, H.A.J., Gielen, W.W., Cools, A.R. and van Rossum, J.M. (1974) Arch. int. Pharmacodyn., 209, 324-331.
31. Kebabian, J.W., Calne, D.B. (1979) Nature, 277, 93-96.
32. Bennett, J.P. and Snyder, S.H. (1970) Mol. Pharmacol., 12, 373-389.
33. Closse, A. and Hauser, D. (1976) Life Sci., 19, 1851-1854.
34. Papp, R.H., Hawkins, H.B., Share, N.N. and Wang, S.C. (1966) J. Pharmacol. exp. Ther., 154, 333-338.
35. Share, N.N., Chai, C.Y. and Wang, S.C. (1965) J. Pharmacol. exp. Ther., 147, 416-421.
36. Loew, D.M., Vigouret, J.M. and Jaton, A.L. (1979) in Dopaminergic Ergot Derivatives and Motor Function, Calne, D.P. and Fuxe, K. ed., Wenner-Green Symposium (in press) Pergamon Press, New York.
37. Boismare, F. and Micheli, L. (1974) J. Pharmacol. (Paris), 5, 221-230.
38. Cahn, J. and Borzeix, M.G. (1978) Gerontology (Basel) Suppl.1, 34-42.

39.Gygax, P., Wiernsperger, N., Meier-Ruge, W. and Baumann, T. (1978) Gerontology (Basel), 24, Suppl.1, 14-22.
40.Boulu, R.G. (1978) Gerontology (Basel), 24, Suppl.1, 139-149.
41.Brown, R., Davis, J.N. and Carlsson, A. (1973) J. Pharm. Pharmac., 25, 412-
   414.
42.Brown, R., Kehr, W. and Carlsson, A. (1975) Brain Res. 85, 491-504.
43.Jäggi, U.H. and Loew, D.M. (1976) Experientia, 32, 779.
44.Boismare, F., Le Pincin, M. Le François, J. (1978) Gerontology (Basel), 24,
   Suppl.1, 6-13.
45.Züger, P.E., Vigouret, J.M. and Loew, D.M. (1978) Experientia, 34, 637-639.
46.Aghajanian, G. (1976) Neuropharmacology, 15, 521-528.
47.Jaton, A.L., Vigouret, J.M., Loew, D.M. (1979) Effects of Hydergine and
   bromocriptine on maze aquisition in rats. Experientia, 35, (in press)
48.Richardson, B.P. (1978) in Action on Ageing, Davison, A.N., Hood, N.A. ed.,
   MCS Consultants, Turnbridge Wells, UK, pp. 32-33.
49.Vigouret, J.M., Jaton, A.L. and Loew, D.M. (1979) Increased senisitivity
   after repeated administration of ergot derivatives to rats. Experientia, 35
   (in press).
50.Ungerstedt, U. (1971) Acta physiol. scand. Suppl. 367, 69-73.
51.Bürki, H.R. (1974) Arzneim. Forsch. (Drug Res.), 24, 983-984.
52.Sayers, A.C. and Kleinlogel, H. (1974) Arzneim. Forsch. (Drug Res.) 24,
   981-983.
53.Martres, M.P., Constentin, J., Baudry, M., Marcais, H., Protais, P. and
   Schwartz, S.C. (1977) Brain Res. 136, 319-337.

CONTROLLED STUDIES WITH DIHYDROERGOTOXINE IN SENILE CEREBRAL INSUFFICIENCY

ALBERT FANCHAMPS, M.D.
Medical Counsel, Pharmaceutical Research and Development, Sandoz Ltd, Basle

INTRODUCTION

Dihydroergotoxine (Hydergine ®, DHTX) was introduced in 1949 as an adreno-sympatholytic drug mainly for use in the treatment of hypertension and peripheral vascular disorders. As an antihypertensive drug, it was rapidly superseded by more active products, and several years were to elapse before its main indication today, senile brain impairment, emerged little by little, in the light of clinical experience.

These early clinical observations are to be found in the literature (Table 1), but it should be remembered that in the fifties the technique of rigorously controlled studies had not yet been developed, so that these trials do not provide incontrovertible evidence of the value of the treatment, even though the results obtained were largely positive.

TABLE 1

EFFECTS OF DIHYDROERGOTOXINE IN SENILE DEMENTIA - "HISTORICAL" STUDIES

Strauss[58,59] 1951/54	Germany	improvement in 37/51 cases	
Benton et al.[8] 1951	USA	DHTX (>) placebo	
Popkin[44,45] 1952/56	USA	400 cases/3 years, majority improved	
Labecki & Busby[31] 1954	USA	DHTX > placebo	
Forster et al.[12] 1955	USA	DHTX = placebo	
Hollister[26] 1955	USA	DHTX > placebo	
Hofstatter et al.[24] 1956	USA	DHTX > { nicotinyl alcohol + pentetrazol / placebo }	
Kaiser & Tschabitscher[28] 1956	Austria	improvement	
Orma[40] 1956	Finland	DHTX > placebo	

> : better than   (>): marginally better than   =: no different from

At that time it was believed that senile dementia was essentially due to cerebro-vascular insufficiency of atherosclerotic origin, and the first clinical pharmacological studies thus sought to establish an effect of dihydro-ergotoxine on cerebral blood flow.

The results obtained were inconsistent and to some extent disappointing (Table 2). However, it would be wrong to lend too much significance to these studies, since it is now well established that in senile dementia cerebro-vascular disturbances and atherosclerosis do not in fact play the pre-eminent role attributed to them a few years ago. Metabolic disturbances of the brain cells are more important and are the main point of attack of drugs employed today to treat senile cerebral insufficiency.

TABLE 2

DIHYDROERGOTOXINE AND CEREBRAL BLOOD FLOW

Authors	Patients	Method	Route of Admin.	Results
McCall et al.[33] 1953	normal and pre-eclamptic females	Kety-Schmidt	i.m.	O
Krauland-Steinbereithner[29] 1958	Schizophrenia Senile cerebral insufficiency	Kety-Schmidt	i.m.	where initial values were low, blood flow and oxygen consumption normalised
Heyck[22] 1959	cerebro-vascular insufficiency	Kety-Schmidt		where initial values were low, blood flow and oxygen consumption increased
Géraud et al.[15] 1963	cerebro-vascular insufficiency	^{85}Kr	i.v.	blood flow and oxygen consumption increased
Gottstein[17] 1963	cerebro-vascular insufficiency	Kety-Schmidt	i.v.	O
McHenry et al.[35] 1971	cerebro-vascular disorders	rCBF ^{133}Xe	i.m.	O

O = no detectable effects

The techniques available for studying brain metabolism in man are limited, since it is not usually possible to obtain brain biopsies, and other invasive methods cannot be employed readily in human subjects. Apart from measurement of the cerebral circulation which is most probably of minor relevance in testing the activity of geriatric medicaments, the only clinical pharmacological methods available today are:

- evaluation of symptoms by means of rating scales
- measurement of performance by means of psychometric tests
- electroencephalogram analysis.

RATING SCALES

The use of clinical rating scales in geriatrics is not new, but until recently they were often applied somewhat unsystematically: some investigators attempted to employ scales designed for other disorders (generally psychiatric), and other investigators drew up lists of symptoms rather haphazardly, without codifying their evaluation.

The first studies of dihydroergotoxine using rating scales were carried out in Europe (mostly in Germany) from 1963 onwards, and elicited mainly positive results (Table 3). However, due to the incongruous nature of the symptoms taken into account and to the fact that they were usually not well defined, no clear demonstration of the treatment's effectiveness could be derived from these investigations. A more systematic method was developed by Venn[62] in 1968. His first concern was to draw up a list of the symptoms of senile dementia cited most frequently in the geriatric literature. In this way he arrived at a list of 38 symptoms which may be classified in 4 categories:

- impairment of cognitive functions
- changes in mood and behaviour
- impaired ability to cope with daily living activities
- physical complaints such as dizziness, fatigue and loss of appetite, not due to a concomitant disease.

This list was tested in a number of double-blind studies in which dihydroergotoxine was compared with placebo in approximately 200 patients (Banen[5], Ditch et al.[10], Pelz[43], Triboletti & Ferri[61]). After evaluation, only those symptoms consistently present in at least 60% of the patients were retained for the final rating scale, which is known in the English-speaking world as the "Sandoz Clinical Assessment Geriatric Scale" or SCAG (Table 4).

TABLE 3

DIHYDROERGOTOXINE - FIRST EUROPEAN STUDIES USING RATING SCALES

Authors	Country	Type of trial	Target symptoms improved/total
Sander-Treske[53] 1963	Germany	open	6 / 7
Orth[41] 1965	Germany	open	10 / 11
Michaelis[37] 1966	Germany	open	3 / 7
Hoffmeister[23] 1967	Germany	open	6 / 7
De la Revilla & Alvarado[49] 1967	Spain	DHTX/pl	6 / 9
Schnell & Oswald[54] 1967	Germany	a) open b) DHTX/pl	a) 8 / 8 b) 3 / 7 psychometric tests
Arrigo & Mille[1] 1969	Italy	DHTX/pl	8 / 11
Gérin[14] 1969	Belgium	DHTX/pl	13 / 28
Grill & Broicher[18] 1969	Germany	DHTX/pl	9 / 11
Seus*[55] 1969	Germany	DHTX/pl	9 / 16 5 / 11 psychometric tests

pl = placebo
*   Detailed results in Heiss et al.[19]

The SCAG includes a precise definition and clear instructions for evaluation on a 7-point scale for each of the 18 target symptoms and the overall impression.

The validity of the SCAG was tested by Shader et al.[56]. They confirmed in a group of 51 patients over age 65 that the scale permits the sharp, statistically significant differentiation between 4 subgroups of subjects for all the symptoms (except for dizziness, which occurred infrequently in their patients):

- normal elderly people

- elderly people with minimal to mild early senile deterioration compatible with independent living

- patients with primary affective disorders, generally of the depressive type

- patients with marked to severe senile dementia.

TABLE 4

SCAG - LIST OF SYMPTOMS

---

1. Confusion	10. Irritability
2. Mental alertness	11. Hostility
3. Impairment of recent memory	12. Bothersome
4. Disorientation	13. Indifference to surroundings
5. Mood depression	14. Unsociability
6. Emotional lability	15. Uncooperativeness
7. Self-care	16. Fatigue
8. Anxiety	17. Appetite (Anorexia)
9. Motivation, initiative	18. Dizziness
	19. Overall impression of patient

The SCAG was found to be more suited for geriatric patients than another scale widely employed in the United States, the Mental Status Examination Record (MSER). In another part of their study, Shader et al.[56] demonstrated a good correlation between the SCAG scores assigned to eight patients by 4 different raters. They conclude that the SCAG is a valid and reliable research instrument, possessing an adequate power of discrimination.

So far, results from sixteen controlled trials employing the SCAG which were performed in the USA have been evaluated. Dihydroergotoxine was compared either with placebo or with papaverine preparations, in parallel groups of patients. (In pilot trials employing a cross-over design, results were found to be obscured by a carry-over effect.) The duration of treatment was three to twelve months.

Selection of the patients is an important factor: a therapeutic effect is difficult to demonstrate in patients suffering from very mild forms of the disease, while very advanced forms do not respond to any treatment. Experience has shown that suitable patients should have at least the first seven symptoms of the SCAG with a score between 3 (mild) and 5 (moderate); at least two of

200

these symptoms should have a score of 5.

TABLE 5

CONTROLLED US STUDIES USING THE SCAG SCALE - DIHYDROERGOTOXINE-PLACEBO

Authors	No. of cases		Duration (months)	Number of symptoms responding better to DHTX with:		Overall impression in favour of DHTX
	DHTX	Pl		Sign.diff. ($p < 0.05$)	Trend ($p > 0.05$)	
Jennings[27]	24	26	3	8	9	**
Rao & Norris[47]	29	28	3	9	5	**
Short & Benway[57]	23	26	3	11	5	*
Rodriguez[50]	29	30	3	19	–	**
Winslow[64]	25	25	3	15	4	*
Hollingsworth[25]	25	28	3	10	7	(*)
Linden[32]	26	24	3	16	2	**
Gaitz et al.[13]	23	24	6	12	6	**
Gherondache[16]	28	18	12	10	8	*

**$p < 0.01$ *$p < 0.05$ (*)$p < 0.1$

Nine trials comparing dihydroergotoxine and placebo are summarised in Table 5. In each of these, most of the target symptoms reacted better to dihydroergotoxine than to placebo, the difference being significant in the majority of cases; furthermore, with regard to the overall impression, the difference was either significant ($p < 0.01$ in 5, $p < 0.05$ in 3 trials) or near-significant ($p < 0.1$ in one trial) in favour of dihydroergotoxine.

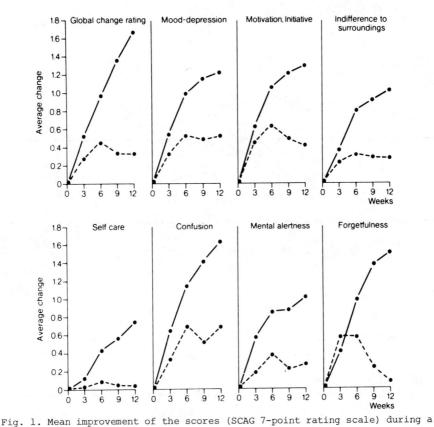

Fig. 1. Mean improvement of the scores (SCAG 7-point rating scale) during a double-blind trial over 12 weeks.
●————●dihydroergotoxine 1 mg t.i.d. in 29 subjects, mean age 79 years
●- - - -●placebo in 28 subjects, mean age 77 years
After Rao and Norris [47] (by permission of the Johns Hopkins University Press).

Figure 1 shows typical time-response curves for eight items of the rating scale: while in the group treated with dihydroergotoxine the target symptoms showed progressive improvement, treatment with placebo afforded initial improvement, which levelled out or declined after 3-6 weeks. The difference between dihydroergotoxine and placebo widened week by week.

Table 6 is a summary of the trials comparing dihydroergotoxine and papaverine preparations which are widely used in the USA for the treatment of senile dementia. Again, the majority of the target symptoms responded better to dihydroergotoxine, although differences were less consistently significant than when dihydroergotoxine was compared with placebo; the overall impression was in each study in favour of dihydroergotoxine, but the difference was statistically significant only in three of the six studies and of borderline significance in another.

TABLE 6

CONTROLLED US STUDIES USING THE SCAG SCALE - DIHYDROERGOTOXINE-PAPAVERINE

Authors	No. of cases		Duration (months)	Number of symptoms responding better to DHTX with:		Overall impression in favour of DHTX
	DHTX	Pl		Sign.diff. (p< 0.05)	Trend (p > 0.05)	
Bazo[7]	33	33	3	4	9	(*)
Rao[46]	20	20	3	1	12	n.s.
Rosen[51]	26	27	3	13	2	**
Winslow[65]	27	26	3	17	1	**
Nelson[39]	25	20	3	14	1	**
Einspruch[11]	21	18	3	6	11	n.s.

**p< 0.01   *p< 0.05   (*) p< 0.1   n.s. p > 0.1

It is interesting to note which symptoms show the most clear-cut and consistent response. Figure 2, which is based on the results of 14 American studies comparing dihydroergotoxine with placebo or papaverine, shows that statistically significant differences in favour of dihydroergotoxine were observed most frequently for the symptoms mood depression, confusion, mental alertness, anxiety and unsociability, while bothersomeness exhibited the least consistent response. Of the 18 symptoms, only 7 were ever reported as responding better to the reference (papaverine in 5 cases and placebo in 2), and each only in one of the 14 trials.

Effect on symptoms in 14 controlled trials (USA)
Ordinate: Number of trials
Abscissa: Level of significance of the difference between Hydergine and the reference
preparation (placebo or papaverine).

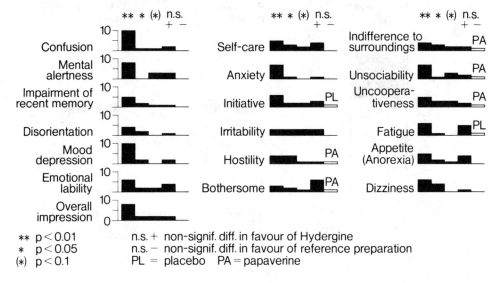

** p<0.01   n.s. + non-signif. diff. in favour of Hydergine
* p<0.05   n.s. − non-signif. diff. in favour of reference preparation
(*) p<0.1   PL = placebo PA = papaverine

Fig. 2. A summary of the results obtained in 14 trials comparing dihydroergotoxine (Hydergine) with placebo (Gaitz et al.[13], Hollingsworth[25], Jennings[27],
Linden[32], Rao and Norris[47], Rodriguez[50], Short and Benway[57], Winslow[64]) or with
papaverine preparations (Bazo[7], Einspruch[11], Nelson[39], Rao[46], Rosen[51],
Winslow[65]).

Another measure of the effectiveness of treatment is the percentage of
patients showing various degrees of improvement. Figure 3 summarises the
results of twelve trials, six comparing dihydroergotoxine with papaverine
and six with placebo. In the patients treated with dihydroergotoxine, an
overall improvement of at least 1 point on the SCAG scale was seen in 68.5%
cases; more than 20% of all patients showed a gain of 3 or more points, this
amounting in clinical terms to a very appreciable improvement. The respective figures are 46% and 7% for papaverine, 44% and 5% for placebo.

204

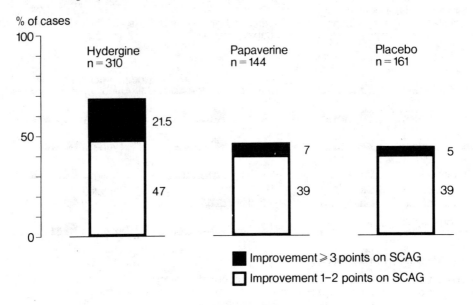

Twelve US studies comparing Hydergine with placebo (6 studies) and Hydergine with papaverine (6 studies) using the SCAG: overall impression – proportion of cases showing improvement.

% of cases

Hydergine n = 310

Papaverine n = 144

Placebo n = 161

■ Improvement ⩾ 3 points on SCAG
□ Improvement 1–2 points on SCAG

Fig. 3. Overall impression in 12 trials comparing dihydroergotoxine with placebo (Hollingsworth[25], Jennings[27], Linden[32], Rao and Norris[47], Rodriguez[50], Winslow[64]) or with papaverine products (Bazo[7], Einspruch [11], Nelson[39], Rao[46], Rosen[51], Winslow[65]).

Based on the American studies done prior to 1973 and a Belgian study by Gérin[14], the US Food & Drug Administration declared dihydroergotoxine effective for the treatment of five symptoms of senile dementia - confusion, depression, unsociability, impairment of self-care and dizziness.

The SCAG was developed in the USA for American patients and geriatricians. A certain latency period elapsed before investigators in other countries applied the scale in its original form or its adaptations in other languages; nevertheless, all the derived rating scales used in recent years have adopted some of its features. Table 7 summarises studies recently carried out in France, Italy, the United Kingdom and Canada with scales akin to the SCAG, the results of which largely confirm those of the American investigators.

TABLE 7

DIHYDROERGOTOXINE - RECENT CONTROLLED TRIALS USING RATING SCALES
CARRIED OUT IN EUROPE AND IN CANADA

Authors	Reference preparation	Number of cases DHTX Ref.		Duration weeks	Number of symptoms responding better to DHTX (sign.)	Comments
Baldoni et al.[4] (Italy)	Nicergoline	20	20	4		equally effective
Bargheon[6] (France)	Placebo	55	54	12	13/17	adaptation of the SCAG
McConnachie[34] (Great Britain)	Placebo	26	26	12	17/22	modified SCAG
Mémin et al.[36] (France)	Nicergoline	26 ✕ 26		2x4		cross over trial equally effective
Rehman[48] (Great Britain)	Placebo	a) 46 ✕ 46		2x8		a) 1st period DHTX > Pl 2nd period DHTX = Pl
		b) 15	15	12	b) 5/10	
Thibault[60] (Canada)	Placebo	22	26	12	13/18	
Paux et al.[42] (France)	Placebo	25	24	12	5/13	abridged SCAG

✕ cross-over design

ELECTROENCEPHALOGRAM

Since the effects of cerebral aging on the electroencephalogram (EEG) are
now well established, it was interesting to ascertain whether the subjective
improvements discernible with the aid of the SCAG or similar rating scales
were accompanied by an objectively demonstrable improvement in the EEG. Apart
from one US study (Wilder and Gonyea[63]), this approach has been taken by
European clinicians (Table 8).

TABLE 8

CONTROLLED TRIALS DIHYDROERGOTOXINE-PLACEBO USING RATING SCALES AND EEG

Authors	Number of cases DHTX Pl		Duration weeks	Number of symptoms responding better to DHTX (sign.)	Correlation between clinical improvement and EEG
Roubicek et al.[52] (Switzerland)	22	22	12	10 / 32	yes
Arrigo et al.[2] (Italy)	10	10	12	5 / 18	yes
Arrigo[3] (Giove & Necchi) (Italy)	15	15	24	6 / 18	yes
Wilder & Gonyea[63] (USA)	16	12	6	9 / 17 (SCAG)	yes
Biel et al.[9] (Germany)	51 cross-over	51	15	4 / 7	yes

Although the EEG was evaluated visually in these first studies, all of them confirmed that a good correlation exists between clinical improvement and the 'rejuvenation' of the EEG, which finds expression mainly in an acceleration of the dominant frequency, an increase in amplitude of the alpha waves and a relative decrease in slow waves. Quantified methods of evaluation make it now possible to detect still more subtle correlations.

In the German study by Herzfeld et al.[20,21], the rating scale and EEG were supplemented by psychometric tests and radiocirculographic measurement of the cerebral circulation time (a decrease in cerebral circulation time denotes an increase in blood flow) (Table 9); the four methods produced evidence of improvement in the group treated with dihydroergotoxine. A parallel improvement of the symptoms - as assessed with the help of a rating scale - and of the cerebral circulation time was also observed in an open study by Mongeau[38] in Canada. Although the study by Kugler et al.[30] did not make use of a clinical rating scale, the other methods employed correspond to those used by Herzfeld[20,21] - except that the EEG was analysed by computer; the study ran for

15 months and was thus able to show the deterioration of the cerebral circulation time in the subjects in the placebo group, which contrasted with the
variable degree of improvement observed in psychometric tests, the EEG and
radio-circulography in those treated with dihydroergotoxine.

TABLE 9

CONTROLLED TRIALS DIHYDROERGOTOXINE-PLACEBO USING PSYCHOMETRIC TESTS, EEG,
RADIO-CIRCULOGRAPHY (AND A RATING SCALE IN ONE STUDY)

Authors	Herzfeld et al.[20,21] (Germany)	Kugler et al.[30] (Germany)
No. of cases DHTX-Pl	33 - 32	60 - 40
Duration	6 weeks	60 weeks
Rating scale: no. symptoms responding better to DHTX/total no.	9 / 14	
Psychometric tests: no. items responding better to DHTX/total no.	5 / 9	7 / 10
Correlation with EEG improvement	yes	yes
Cerebral circulation time	DHTX ↘ Pl =	DHTX ↘ Pl ↗

CONCLUSIONS

   Senile cerebral insufficiency is considered poorly amenable to treatment,
and until ten or so years ago, few studies had furnished convincing evidence
that drugs had any value in this field.

   The papers which have been reviewed show that with the improved design of
clinical rating scales, culminating in the development of the SCAG, it is now
possible to demonstrate the effect of a drug such as dihydroergotoxine and of
differentiating it from placebo or products based on papaverine, in a statistically significant manner.

Single positive studies may not be entirely convincing: it is always possible that an unrecognised bias can have crept in or that owing to special circumstances the results are not generally valid. It is, therefore, desirable to base assessment on several trials carried out according to comparable protocols, but by different investigators in different geographical areas. When most of the results are in agreement, there can be no doubt about their validity.

In the case of dihydroergotoxine, the almost complete agreement of the results obtained using the SCAG and similar rating scales has been additionally corroborated by its consistent effects on the EEG.

SUMMARY

The first controlled trials which demonstrated the value of dihydroergotoxine (Hydergine ®) in the treatment of senile cerebral insufficiency date back to 1951, and clinical rating scales have been used since 1963 in further demonstrations of the effect of the drug. However, only in the last 10 years has a systematic attempt been made to establish a reliable and valid clinical rating scale with a sufficient discriminatory power. This led to the development of the SCAG (Sandoz Clinical Assessment Geriatric Scale). The scale embodies an inventory of 18 target symptoms which the investigator scores according to a 1-7 rating key; its usefulness has been confirmed in a validatory study. So far it has been employed in 16 controlled studies in a total of about 800 cases in the USA; these studies revealed significant differences favouring dihydroergotoxine over placebo (10 studies), or significant differences or at least trends favouring dihydroergotoxine over papaverine (6 studies). The symptoms reacting most consistently to dihydroergotoxine are confusion, mental alertness, mood depression, anxiety and unsociability. Geriatricians outside the United States have not usually adopted the SCAG in its original form, but numerous investigators in the United Kingdom, Germany, Canada, France, Italy and Switzerland have made use of it in developing their own scales, which have furnished comparable results. In a number of European trials, rating scales have been used in conjunction with electroencephalography and sometimes also with psychometric tests and cerebral radio-circulography; these various methods have borne out the beneficial effects of treatment with dihydroergotoxine, and provided evidence of correlations between rating scales and more objective physical parameters as a basis for drug evaluation.

REFERENCES

1. Arrigo, A., Mille, T. (1969). Sull'impiego del Visergil nella profilassi e terapia della sclerosi cerebrale. Neuropsichiatria 35 (1).

2. Arrigo, A., Braun, P., Kauchtschischwili, G.M., Moglia, A., Tartara, A. (1973). Influence of Treatment on Symptomatology and Correlated Electroence-phalographic (EEG) Changes in the Aged. Curr. ther. Res. 15, 417-426.

3. Arrigo, A. (1975). Influencia de la Hydergina sobre los trastornos cerebro-vasculares seniles y su correlación con los cambios en el electroencefalo-grama. Invest. Médica Internacional 2, Supl. (1), 45-60.

4. Baldoni, E., Serenthà, P., Cuttin, S., Galetti, G. (1971). L'azione tera-peutica della nimergolina negli anziani arteriosclerotici con insufficienza cerebrale vascolare. Gazz. int. Med. Chir. 76, 965-974.

5. Banen, D.M. (1972). An ergot Preparation (Hydergine) for Relief of Symptoms of Cerebrovascular Insufficiency. J. Amer. Geriatr. Soc. 20 (1), 22-24.

6. Bargheon, J. (1973). Etude en double insu de l'Hydergine chez le sujet âgé. Nouv. Presse méd. 2, 2053-2055.

7. Bazo, A.J. (1973). An Ergot Alkaloid Preparation (Hydergine) Versus Papa-verine in Treating Common Complaints of the Aged: Double-Blind Study. J. Amer. Geriatr. Soc. 21 (2), 63-71.

8. Benton, J.G., Brown, H., Rinzler, S.H. (1951). Objective Evaluation of Physical and Drug Therapy in the Rehabilitation of the Hemiplegic Patient. Am. Heart J. 42, 719-732.

9. Biel, M.-L., Seus, R., Struppler, A. (1976). Medikamentöse Therapie des hirn-organischen Psychosyndroms im Alter. Med. Klin. 71, 2177-2184.

10. Ditch, M., Kelly, F.J., Resnick, O. (1971). An Ergot Preparation (Hydergine) in the Treatment of Cerebrovascular Disorders in the Geriatric Patient: A Double-Blind Study. J. Amer. Geriatr. Soc. 19, 208-217.

11. Einspruch, B.C. (1976). Helping to Make the Final Years Meaningful for the Elderly Residents of Nursing Homes. Dis. nerv. Syst. 37, 439-442.

12. Forster, W., Schultz, S., Henderson, A.L. (1955). Combined Hydrogenated Alkaloids of Ergot in Senile and Arteriosclerotic Psychoses. Geriatr., Minneapolis 10, 26-30.

13. Gaitz, C.M., Varner, R., Overall, J.E. (1977). Pharmacotherapy for Organic Brain Syndrome in Late Life. Evaluation of an Ergot Derivative vs. Placebo. Arch. gen. Psychiat. 34, 839-845.

14. Gérin, J. (1969). Symptomatic Treatment of Cerebrovascular Insufficiency with Hydergine. Curr. ther. Res. 11, 539-546.

15. Géraud, J., Bès, A., Rascol, A., Delpla, M., Marc-Vergnes, J.P. (1963). Mesure du débit sanguin cérébral au krypton 85. Quelques applications physio-pathologiques et cliniques. Rev. Neurol. 108, 542-557.

16. Gherondache, D.N. (1977). Data on file at Sandoz Inc., East Hanover, N.J., USA.

17. Gottstein, U. (1963). Durchblutungsstörungen des Gehirns. Therapiewoche 13, 922-928.

18. Grill, P., Broicher, H. (1969). Zur Therapie der zerebralen Insuffizienz. Deutsch. Med. Wschr. 94, 2429-2435.

19. Heiss, R., Seus, R., Fahrenberg, J. (1971). Eine Studie zur Prüfung der psychodynamischen Wirkung von Dihydroergotoxin. Arzneim.-Forsch. 21, 797-800.

20. Herzfeld, U., Christian, W., Oswald, W.D., Ronge, J., Wittgen, M. (1972). Zur Wirkungsanalyse von Hydergin im Langzeitversuch. Med. Klin. 67, 1118-1125.

21. Herzfeld, U., Christian, W., Ronge, J., Wittgen, M. (1972). Richtgrössen für die Beurteilung der Hirnfunktion nach Langzeittherapie mit Hydergin. Aerztl. Forschg. 26, 215-228.

22. Heyck, H. (1959). Der Einfluss gefässaktiver sympathicolytischer Medikamen-
te auf die Hämodynamik und den Sauerstoffverbrauch des Gehirns bei cerebro-
vasculären Erkrankungen. Messungen mit der Stickoxydulmethode im akuten und
chronischen Versuch. Dtsch. Zschr. Nervenhk. 179, 58-74.

23. Hoffmeister, K. (1967). Klinische Aspekte zur Therapie der Zerebralsklerose.
Med. Klin. 62, 910-912.

24. Hofstatter, L., Ossorio, A., Mandl, B., Kohler, L.H., Busch, A.K., Hyman, A.
(1956). Pharmaceutical Treatment of Patients with Senile Brain Changes.
Arch. Neurol. Psychiatr. (Chicago) 75, 316-322.

25. Hollingsworth, S.W. (1974). Effective Nursing Home Care for Elderly Patients.
Evaluation and Treatment. Scient. Exhibit. Am. Med. Ass., Clin. Conv., Portland, Oregon, Nov. 30 - Dec. 3.

26. Hollister, L.E. (1955). Combined Hydrogenated Alkaloids of Ergot in Mental
and Nervous Disorders Associated with Old Age. Dis. nerv. Syst. 16, 259-262.

27. Jennings, W.C. (1972). An Ergot Alkaloid Preparation (Hydergine) Versus Placebo for Treatment of Symptoms of Cerebrovascular Insufficiency: Double-
Blind Study. J. Amer. Geriatr. Soc. 20, 407-412.

28. Kaiser, G., Tschabitscher, H. (1956). Erfahrungen mit Hydergin in der Behandlung zerebraler Durchblutungsstörungen im höheren Alter. Wiener klin.
Wochenschr. 9, 150-154.

29. Krauland-Steinbereithner, F. (1958). Untersuchungen über Hirndurchblutung
und Hirnstoffwechsel an einem psychiatrischen Krankengut. Wien. Zschr.
Nervenhk. 15, 158-169.

30. Kugler, J., Oswald, W.D., Herzfeld, U., Seus, R., Pingel, J., Welzel, D.
(1978). Langzeittherapie altersbedingter Insuffizienzerscheinungen des Gehirns. Dtsch. med. Wschr. 103, 456-462.

31. Labecki, T.D., Busby, C.L. (1954). Dihydrogenated Ergot Derivatives in
Cerebral Arteriosclerosis. J. Geront. 9, 485-486.

32. Linden, M.E. (1975). Retirement and the Elderly Patient. Problems and Practical Therapy. Scient. Exhibit./ Amer. Geriatr. Soc., 32nd Ann. Meeting,
Miami Beach, Florida, April 16-17.

33. McCall, M.L.,Taylor, H.W. (1953). The Action of Hydergine on the Circulation
and Metabolism of the Brain in Toxemia of Pregnancy. Amer. J. med. Sci. 226,
537-540.

34. McConnachie, R.W. (1973). A clinical Trial Comparing "Hydergine" with Placebo in the Treatment of Cerebrovascular Insufficiency in Elderly Patients.
Curr. med. Res. Opin. 1, 463-468.

35. McHenry, L.C., Jaffe, M.E., Kawamura, J., Goldberg, H.I. (1971). Hydergine
Effect on Cerebral Circulation in Cerebrovascular Disease. J. neurol. Sci.
13, 475-481.

36. Mémin, Y., Najean Hueber, E. (1973). Etude à double-insu selon une échelle
d'appréciation quantitative d'un traitement des troubles vasculaires céré-
braux chroniques. Entretiens de Bichat, Vol. Thérap.: Expansion Scientif.
Française, Paris, 239-242.

37. Michaelis, U. (1966). Zur Symptomatik und Therapie der Zerebralsklerose in
der Praxis. Ther. der Gegenw. 105, 1593-1600.

38. Mongeau, B. (1974). The effect of Hydergine on the Transit Time of Cerebral
Circulation in Diffuse Cerebral Insufficiency. Europ. J. clin. Pharmacol. 7,
169-175.

39. Nelson, J.J. (1975). Relieving Selected Symptoms of the Elderly. Geriatrics
30, 133-139, 142.

40. Orma, E.J. (1956). Hydrogenated Ergotalkaloids (Hydergine) in the Treatment
of Geriatric Postural Dizziness. Ann. Med. Int. Fenn. 45, 39-44.

41. Orth, H. (1965). Zur Therapie der Zerebralsklerose in der täglichen Praxis. Med. Klin. 60, 266-269.
42. Paux, G., Boismare, F., Delaunay, P. (1975). Etude en double aveugle de l'Hydergine chez le sujet âgé. Nouv. Presse méd. 4, 2529.
43. Pelz, D.S. (1968). Hydergine Versus Placebo. Data on file at Sandoz Inc., East Hanover, N.J., USA.
44. Popkin, R.J. (1952). The Hydrogenated Alkaloids of Ergot in Geriatrics. Amer. Pract. 3, 532-535.
45. Popkin, R.J. (1956). The Hydrogenated Alkaloids of Ergot (Hydergine) in Geriatrics - Follow Up Study. Amer. Pract. 7, 1594-1597.
46. Rao, D.B. (1973). Double-Blind Study of Hydergine Versus Papaverine in the Treatment of Cerebrovascular Insufficiency in the Elderly. Data on file at Sandoz Inc., East Hanover, N.J., USA.
47. Rao, D.B., Norris, J.R. (1972). A Double-Blind Investigation of Hydergine in the Treatment of Cerebrovascular Insufficiency in the Elderly. Johns Hopkins Med. J. 130, 317-324.
48. Rehman, S.A. (1973). Two Trials Comparing "Hydergine" with Placebo in the Treatment of Patients Suffering from Cerebrovascular Insufficiency. Curr. med. Res. Opin. 1, 456-462.
49. De la Revilla, L., Alvarado, J.J. (1967). La Hydergina en la Terapeutica Geriatrica. Med. esp. 58, 105-113.
50. Rodriguez, J.M. (1973). A Double-Blind Placebo Controlled Study of Hydergine in the Treatment of Cerebrovascular Insufficiency in the Elderly. Data on file at Sandoz Inc., East Hanover, N.J., USA.
51. Rosen, H.J. (1975). Mental Decline in the Elderly: Pharmacotherapy (Ergot Alkaloids Versus Papaverine). J. Amer. Geriatr. Soc. 23, 169-174.
52. Roubicek, J., Geiger, Ch., Abt, K. (1972). An Ergot Alkaloid Preparation (Hydergine) in Geriatric Therapy. J. Amer. Geriatr. Soc. 20, 222-229.
53. Sander-Treske, R. (1963). Beitrag zur Behandlung sklerotisch bedingter cerebraler Durchblutungsstörungen mit Hydergin. Berl. Med. 14, 207-209.
54. Schnell, R., Oswald, W.D. (1967). Geriatrische Pharmakotherapie des neurasthenischen Syndroms. Aerztl. Forsch. 21, 464-470.
55. Seus, R. (1969). A Model Study on Geriatric Drug Testing under Realistic Practical Conditions. In: 8th International Congress of Gerontology, Washington, D.C. Proceedings, Vol. II, 52.
56. Shader, R.I., Harmatz, J.S., Salzman, C. (1974). A new Scale for Clinical Assessment in Geriatric Populations: Sandoz Clinical Assessment - Geriatric (SCAG). J. Amer. Geriatr. Soc. 22, 107-113.
57. Short, M.J., Benway, M. (1972). Delivery of Mental Health Services to the Elderly ... the State Hospital and the Community. Scient. Exhibit. Amer. Psychiatr. Ass., Dallas, Texas, May 1-5.
58. Strauss, H.L. (1951). Klinische Erfahrungen mit "Hydergin" (CCK 179). Med. Welt 20, 113-115.
59. Strauss, H.L. (1954). Klinische Erfahrungen mit Hydergin. Cardiologia 25, 1-36.
60. Thibault, A. (1974). A Double-Blind Evaluation of "Hydergine" and Placebo in the Treatment of Patients with Organic Brain Syndrome and Cerebral Arteriosclerosis in a Nursing Home. Curr. med. Res. Opin. 2, 482-487.
61. Triboletti, F., Ferri, H. (1969). Hydergine for Treatment of Symptoms of Cerebrovascular Insufficiency. Curr. ther. Res. 11, 609-620.
62. Venn, R.D. (1978). Clinical Pharmacology of Ergot Alkaloids in Senile Cerebral Insufficiency. In: Ergot Alkaloids and Related Compounds. Ed.: Berde, B. and Schild, H.C., Springer-Verlag Berlin, Heidelberg, New York, 533-566.

63. Wilder, B.J., Gonyea, E.F. (1973). The effects of the Dihydrogenated Ergot Alkaloids on Symptoms of Aging. Scient. Exhibit. Amer. Med. Ass. Ann. Conv., New York, N.Y., June 23-27.
64. Winslow, I.E. (1974a). Mental Decline in the Aged: Aspects of Etiology and Therapy. Scient. Exhibit. Amer. Geriatr. Soc. Ann. Meeting, Toronto, Canada, April 17-18.
65. Winslow, I.E. (1974b). The Hospitalized Geriatric Patient. Scient. Exhibit. Amer. Med. Assoc. Meeting, Portland, Oregon, Nov. 30-Dec. 3.

Published 1979 by Elsevier North Holland, Inc.
Nandy, Ed. Geriatric Psychopharmacology

ERGOT ALKALOIDS IN TREATMENT OF GERIATRIC PATIENTS WITH DEMENTIA

CHARLES M. GAITZ, M.D., and JAMES T. HARTFORD, M.D.
  Texas Research Institute of Mental Sciences, Texas Medical Center,
  1300 Moursund, Houston, Texas 77030, USA

Ergot alkaloids have been used to treat patients for hypertension and other
vascular problems, such as migraine, for at least fifty years. In 1949, one of
these products, dihydroergotoxine, was introduced for the treatment of hypertension and peripheral vascular disease. Some years later came the observation
than many elderly patients who also had dementia began to improve while taking
the new drug[1-11]. Physicians began to investigate the efficacy of the ergot
alkaloids in treatment for cognitive impairment and behavioral changes associated with senility. The results of some of these early investigations, summarized in Table 1, led to the hope that ergot alkaloids would provide definitive
treatment for senile dementia[4]. Although this expectation has not been fully
realized, the contention that ergot alkaloids are of benefit to elderly patients with organic brain syndrome continues to be supported by research[12-24].

TABLE 1

EARLY STUDIES ON EFFECTS OF HYDERGINE IN SENILE DEMENTIA

Author	Year	Country	Results
Strauss[1,2]	1951,1954	Germany	Improvement in 74% of cases
Benton et al[3]	1951	USA	Hydergine superior to placebo
Popkin[4,5]	1952,1956	USA	400 cases followed over 3-year period improved and had fewer illnesses
Lambecki and Busby[6]	1954	USA	Hydergine superior to placebo
Hollister[7]	1955	USA	Hydergine superior to placebo
Forster et al[8]	1955	USA	Results equivocal
Orma[9]	1956	Finland	Hydergine superior to placebo
Hofstater et al[10]	1956	USA	Hydergine superior to placebo or pentetrazole and nicotinyl alcohol
Kaiser and Tschabitscher[11]	1956	Austria	Improvement with Hydergine

Some ergot alkaloids are known to have central nervous system effects, and one, dihydroergotoxine (Hydergine), has been investigated extensively in treatment of dementia. Hydergine is a combination of three ergot alkaloids: dihydroergocornine mesylate, dihydroergocristine mesylate, and dihydroergokryptine mesylate. Two other alkaloids, nicergoline (Sermion) and dihydroergonine (DN 16-457), have also been studied, but not as extensively. We will report only on experiences with Hydergine, restricting our discussion to the use of Hydergine for patients who have impaired cognition and other changes attributable to Alzheimer's disease and cerebral vascular disease, not to the many other conditions associated with organic brain syndrome.

RATIONALE FOR TREATMENT

The cognitive impairment and behavioral changes that occur in elderly persons and are presumed to be associated with aging have been called dementia, senile brain disease, organic brain syndrome, and other terms. Until recently, cerebral vascular disease was believed to be the etiology of these conditions. Other causes were known or suspected, but physicians and lay persons usually ascribed these problems to "hardening of the arteries," and treatment was directed at improving cerebral blood flow.

Studies of cerebral circulation have in fact documented that blood flow to the brain of demented patients is diminished and that reduced cerebral circulation and impaired mental ability are related. Further investigations have shown, however, that the pathological lesions in patients with dementia are located in brain cells and are not confined to the blood vessels. Diminution of cerebral blood flow probably occurs secondarily to disease processes that affect brain tissue rather than being the result of primary vascular disease.

Because of this, efforts to improve cerebral blood flow do not alleviate the major problem in most cases of dementia, and drugs presumed to have only a vasodilating effect have limited application in treating patients with organic brain syndrome. In a recent review, Yesavage et al[25] also came to this conclusion. Most elderly patients diagnosed as demented have Alzheimer's disease; that is, their brain cells have undergone neuropathologic changes. Their cognitive impairment and behavioral changes are probably related to brain-cell malfunction, which is accompanied by corresponding decline in blood flow[26-27]. In some demented persons, however, pathologists have demonstrated a combination of parenchymal and vascular disease; in a smaller proportion of these patients, they have noted only vascular disease[28]. Alzheimer's disease was at one time believed to be a presenile condition, but now there seems to be no clinical or anatomical basis for distinguishing between presenile and senile dementia.

Although much remains to be learned about brain physiology, clinicians are probably on target when they treat patients with Alzheimer's disease for primary brain-cell pathology. Circulatory changes may be associated with the condition, but they are secondary. Appropriate therapy should be directed to restoring relatively inactive brain cells to an active functional state, rather than concentrating treatment on such secondary changes as diminished cerebral blood flow.

Neurophysiologists have demonstrated that several brain systems operate simultaneously and that these systems interact; whether the intermediary steps are biochemical, biophysical or electrical, it may be assumed that a change in one system will affect another. The discovery of a definitive treatment may be delayed until we begin to unravel the mysteries of the human brain. We do not know whether dementia associated with vascular disease requires a different treatment than dementia associated with Alzheimer's disease. Nor do we know precisely how nutrition, past and present, or psychological factors influence mental status. We acknowledge the limitations of applying experimental data on these conditions to the treatment of human beings.

ASSESSING METHODS

Serious limitations are inherent in evaluating the efficacy of any modality in the treatment of dementia. Brain biopsies and other invasive techniques could contribute much valuable information, but they present a definite risk and meet with patient resistance. Consequently, they can rarely be incorporated in a scientifically valid protocol. Isolated opportunities for study of human subjects before death arise, but the information thus obtained usually cannot be controlled, follow-up observations are lacking, and the significance of the findings is difficult to evaluate. Noninvasive techniques like skull x-rays and computed axial tomography are more useful in diagnosis than for evaluating treatment. Cerebral vascular dynamics may be monitored with little inconvenience to the patient and the technique is relatively safe, but the information obtained has little value for understanding cerebral metabolic functions. Electroencephalographic recordings are influenced by many factors, making it difficult to correlate abnormal findings with anatomic sites or metabolic phenomena.

Because the techniques just mentioned for evaluation of treatment have inherent weaknesses, researchers often must rely on rating scales as a means of measuring change. Rating scales, of course, are also subject to criticism, not only because there may be a lack of patients' cooperation, but also there may be considerable variation of opinion among the raters' interpretation of the items being rated and assigning scores on the basis of clinical judgment.

Selecting tests to rate behavior and cognition is complicated. Tests that are sensitive enough to detect mild dementia may be too demanding or too sensitive to measure improvement in patients with a severe dementia; tests which could be used to rate patients with a severe dementia may not be sensitive enough for use with patients whose mental impairment is relatively mild. Furthermore, many of the tests that are available have been standardized for use with young and middle-aged populations, and the tests may be irrelevant or invalid for older, impaired patients[29-32].

Advances in psychopharmacology emphasized the need for a reliable instrument to evaluate drug therapy. Early investigators had simply listed symptoms which they considered to be particularly relevant to the study of dementia, then rated changes brought on by drug treatment on a more or less personally determined standard. Such approaches rarely provided reliable data.

To overcome some of these impediments to valid evaluations of drug therapy, Venn developed a scale now known as the Sandoz Clinical Assessment Geriatric Scale (SCAG). The SCAG items were selected from a list of symptoms most commonly observed in elderly patients. A seven-point rating system is used to indicate the degree of severity of each symptom. Shader et al[33] confirmed the reliability of the instrument in distinguishing four groups of elderly persons: A normal group, patients who have primarily affective disorders, those who are minimally demented, and those who are markedly demented. The symptoms rated are the following:

Confusion	Hostility
Mental Alertness	Bothersome
Impairment of Recent Memory	Indifference to Surroundings
Disorientation	Unsociability
Mood Depression	Uncooperativeness
Emotional Lability	Fatigue
Self-Care	Appetite (Anorexia)
Anxiety	Dizziness
Motivation Initiative	Overall Impression of Patient
Irritability	

CLINICAL STUDIES

At least twenty-five published studies have noted mild to moderate improvement when Hydergine was used to treat elderly persons with symptoms of cogni-

tive impairment and behavioral disturbances, the symptoms associated with dementia in elderly persons. In spite of this, many investigators share the senti-
ment expressed in the Medical Letter:[34] "There is no convincing evidence that
dihydrogenated ergot alkaloids are effective for treatment of idiopathic cerebral dysfunction." Many clinicians are equally pessimistic.

While it is true that many of these studies may be criticized for sampling
and other methodological weaknesses, an overview of the reports in the literature supports the contention that ergot alkaloids may be beneficial. But it is
impossible on the basis of these reports to predict how a particular patient
will respond. The following brief review of clinical studies reveals some of
the difficulties in evaluating results across studies because of variations in
the selection of patients, the dosage given, the duration of treatment, and the
severity of disorder.

Forster et al[8] investigated the effects of Hydergine in a sample of fifteen
inpatients whose psychotic condition was associated with a history of cerebral
vascular disease and senile psychosis. No significant improvement in the treatment group compared with a placebo group was noted, but the dosage given did
not exceed 1.5 mg per day. The low dosage may have been a factor in the poor
response to treatment.

Hollister[7] reported a double-blind study of twenty-six patients whose dementia was attributed to arteriosclerosis, senile brain disease, alcoholism, syphilis, and schizophrenia. In this etiologically mixed group, one patient on placebo and six patients on Hydergine improved marginally, and two of the Hydergine
group improved greatly. Patients were observed for nine weeks and dosage was
gradually reduced from 8.0 mg to 4.0 mg per day. Though the dosage seemed
adequate, the diagnoses of patients in this study varied considerably and the
duration of treatment was brief.

Ten other double-blind studies[12-21] compared Hydergine and placebo. A dosage
of 3.0 mg per day was used in eight studies[12-17,20,21] and 4.5 mg per day was
the dosage in the other two[18,19]. Eight[12-19] of the ten studies lasted for
twelve weeks and the other two[20,21] were sixteen and twenty-four weeks long.
Patients with diagnoses of cerebral arteriosclerosis or senile deterioration
were included, while those with possible causes of dementia were excluded. In
each of these studies the group treated with Hydergine improved significantly
compared to the group treated with placebo. The degree of improvement and the
symptoms affected, however, varied from one study to another.

In an open study involving 400 ambulatory patients, Popkin[5] noted that patients taking Hydergine "did far better than expected for an ill and aging

group." Using global ratings, he followed the patients for a period of eighteen months to three years. In contrast, in a double-blind study, Soni and Soni[35] reported a gradual improvement in patients taking Hydergine up to twelve weeks, after which the researchers noted a "demonstrable loss of improvement" over a nine-month period. In other double-blind studies, Novo et al[20] observed patients for sixteen weeks and noted no tendencies to relapse; Gaitz et al[21] noted little difference in improvement in the treatment and placebo groups until after twelve weeks of therapy, but during the next twelve weeks, significant differences favoring Hydergine became obvious. The treatment responses in the latter studies were characterized by gradual, modest changes that accumulated over the entire treatment period. Although the results are generally positive, these longer trials do not provide answers to questions about the value of administering Hydergine over an extended period of time.

In still other studies[22,23,24], the effectiveness of Hydergine and Papaverine was compared. The Hydergine-treated groups showed significantly greater improvement than did the Papaverine-treated groups.

The data from these studies do not give a clear answer to the question about whether Hydergine is more effective in relieving some symptoms more than others. To answer some of the questions about qualitative aspects of change, we examined the results of eight double-blind studies[14-21] that were roughly comparable. Each study had compared Hydergine with placebo. Patients with dementia were excluded unless the etiology was cerebral vascular disease or Alzheimer's disease; the patients received at least 3.0 mg of Hydergine per day, and they were observed for at least twelve weeks. For our purposes, improvement was accepted as significant if the investigator had reported improvement in Hydergine-treated group compared to the placebo-treated group at $p < .05$. The SCAG rating scale was used in two studies, and some comparable items were rated in the same manner in the other six studies. The results are summarized in Table 2.

Inspection of Table 2 shows that significant improvement was reported in at least one study for each one of the eighteen items on the SCAG scale. Two-thirds of the studies reported improvement in mental allertness, anxiety, depression, confusion, and orientation. Half of the studies reported improvement in these five items and also five others; impairment of motivation-initiative, hostility, dizziness, impaired recent memory and emotional lability. Significant improvement was noted in some of the studies on each of the other eight individual items, but the number of studies reporting improvement was less than half.

TABLE 2

RESULTS OF DOUBLE-BLIND STUDIES USING ITEMS OF THE SCAG SCALE
TO COMPARE GROUPS OF PATIENTS TREATED WITH HYDERGINE AND PLACEBO

SCAG Item	Number of studies rating comparable item	Number and percent of studies reporting significant improvement with Hydergine ($p < .05$)
1. Mental alertness	5	4 (80%)
2. Anxiety	4	3 (75%)
3. Depression	8	6 (75%
4. Confusion	6	4 (66.6%)
5. Orientation	3	2 (66.6%)
6. Motivation-Initiative	7	4 (57%)
7. Hostility	6	3 (50%)
8. Dizziness	8	4 (50%)
9. Impaired recent memory	6	3 (50%)
10. Emotional lability	6	3 (50%)
11. Irritability	7	3 (42%)
12. Uncooperativeness	6	2 (33%)
13. Unsociability	7	2 (28%)
14. Fatigue	7	2 (28%)
15. Appetite	7	2 (28%)
16. Self-care	7	2 (28%)
17. Indifference	8	2 (25%)
18. Bothersomeness	4	1 (25%)

Comparisons of the results of one study with another showed some trends, but no precise patterns of symptom improvement could be delineated. None of the studies reported improvement in all of the items. The number of items improved ranged from three to fifteen in these eight studies. Because there were variations between these studies in total number of items rated, number of patients evaluated, and other differences, one can only conclude that there appears to be a trend suggesting that Hydergine-treated patients when compared to placebo-treated groups are more likely to experience an alleviation of symptoms.

Overall[21] examined the data from one study using a factor analysis technique He derived four composite factors which he labeled as indicated below. He noted the redundancy in some of the individual SCAG items, but found that the composite factors function independently. Improved mood, for instance, was not a halo effect of improved cognition or decreased withdrawal. The following shows the percentage of the eight studies referred to previously reporting improvement on the individual items comprising the four factors:

Agitation/Irritability
Emotional lability - 50%
Hostility - 50%
Irritability - 42%
Uncooperativeness - 33%
Bothersomeness - 25%

Mood Depression
Mood depression - 75%
Anxiety - 75%
Dizziness - 50%
Appetite (lack of) - 28%
Fatigue - 28%

Cognitive Dysfunction
Confusion - 66.6%
Mental alertness (lack of) - 66.6%
Disorientation - 66.6%
Impairment of recent memory - 50%
Disorientation - 28%

Withdrawal
Motivation-initiative
(deficit) - 57%
Unsociability - 28%
Indifference to
surroundings - 25%

Overall's[21] analysis of the data from a single study indicated that within the factors, the variables grouped under cognitive dysfunction were the most frequently improved, followed by those related to mood depression. The results from the eight studies we inspected indicate essentially the same pattern. We must make clear, however, that we have not taken the raw data from the studies and subjected this data to factor analyses and computations. The data suggests that more studies reported improvement in the items comprising the cognitive dysfunction factor and mood depression factor than the other two factors.

DOSAGE AND ADMINISTRATION

The currently approved dosage of Hydergine in the United States ranges from 0.5 mg to 3.0 mg daily in divided dosages. This is lower than dosages employed in Europe, which range as high as 12.0 mg daily. The efficacy and safety of a total of 6.0 mg per day in divided doses is currently under investigation in the United States. Our review of clinical studies suggests that 3.0 mg daily is a minimum dose.

Another important aspect of administering the drug is its apparent delayed onset of action. Some years ago, Hollister[36] stated that further treatment is unwarranted if no improvement occurs in six weeks. Sathananthan[37] recommended a trial period of eight to twelve weeks, and Gaitz[21] found that patients often required at least twelve weeks to benefit from the drug and cautioned against discontinuing it prematurely. Novo et al[20] noted that maximal improvement was observed by twelve weeks and that little further improvement occurred by sixteen weeks. It seems reasonable to say, therefore, that treatment should be maintained for twelve to sixteen weeks before Hydergine treatment is discontinued.

SIDE EFFECTS

Side effects of Hydergine are rare and mild, and they recede rapidly when the dosage is lowered or the drug discontinued. With sublingual administration, gastric disturbances, transient nausea, headache, and sublingual irritation have been reported. In a trial with eight patients taking 1.5 mg three times a day, Cayley et al[38] reported three cases of sinus bradycardia of 40 beats per minute. When the medication was discontinued, the patients' pulses returned to normal within 48 hours. Kapoor[39] reported an incident of vasospastic angiitis of the right ring finger in a 52-year-old man taking "one tablet" of Hydergine twice a day for headache. The symptoms disappeared within 20 hours of stopping medication.

Hydergine is now available in oral tablet form. There are no reports in the literature on side effects when the drug is administered in this form.

INDICATIONS FOR PRESCRIBING HYDERGINE

The 1979 edition of Physician's Desk Reference[40] states that Hydergine is

> indicated for the treatment of selected symptoms in elderly patients. Short-term clinical studies have demonstrated modest improvement in levels of performance of self-care and such symptoms as mood depression, confusion, unsociability, and dizziness. These symptoms are of unknown etiology and are not specific to any age group or disease. However, to date, only short-term studies conducted with elderly patients have been reported.

Based on our own clinical experience and a review of the literature, it seems that patients with Alzheimer's disease represent the group of patients who should be given a trial with Hydergine. We do not know if Hydergine is as useful in treating dementia associated with cerebral vascular disease. Use of Hydergine to relieve symptoms, without considering etiology, places an unfair burden of proving efficacy on the agent. Hydergine may have a place in treating elderly persons who have symptoms associated with other etiologies, but this has not been demonstrated in the studies reported in the literature.

The clinical picture of dementia in elderly persons is associated with many etiologies, and many of these conditions respond to appropriate treatment. Systemic diseases, vitamin deficiencies, adverse reactions to drugs, psychiatric

222

disorders, subdural hematomas, brain tumors, are some of the reversible causes of dementia that improve with more or less specific treatment.

There is an issue of credibility in using a medication such as Hydergine as a panacea for everything that ails old people. Studies comparing Hydergine with other medications considered to be effective in treating anxiety, depression, and psychosis have not been done. More research will have to be done to determine whether or not Hydergine effects will be useful in treating patients with a variety of symptoms and etiologies. When these are done, we will know that Hydergine is or is not effective in treating dementia associated with vascular disease and alcoholism, for example, or as an adjunct in treating dementias associated with systemic disorders.

SUMMARY

Clinical trials comparing Hydergine versus placebo or Hydergine versus Papaverine for the treatment of organic brain disease in late life have rather consistently shown some statistical improvement favoring Hydergine. Many questions are unanswered, and these relate to such fundamental issues as dosage, duration of treatment necessary to achieve and maintain benefits, and selection of patients most likely to benefit. Our interpretation of research reports leads us to believe that patients with Alzheimer's disease are candidates for treatment with this agent. Common sense would suggest that patients with mild to moderate symptoms are more likely to improve than those with severe forms of the illness. We believe also that to obtain good results, patients need to be treated for several months and at least at the dosage level currently approved.

The results of studies reported thus far are encouraging, especially when compared with results of other available therapies. More investigation is needed to determine more precisely the drug's mode of action, rationale for treatment, and the characteristics of patients most likely to respond to treatment with Hydergine.

REFERENCES

1. Strauss, H L (1951) Klinische erfahrungen mit "Hydergin" (CCK 179). Med. Welt 20:113-115.
2. Strauss, H L (1954) Klinische erfahrungen mit Hydergin. Cardiologia 25:1-36.
3. Benton, J G, Brown, H, Rinzler, S H (1951) Objective evaluation of physical and drug therapy in the rehabilitation of the hemiplegic patient. Am. Heart J. 42:719-732.

4. Popkin, R J (1952) The hydrogenated alkaloids of ergot (Hydergine) in geriatrics. Am. Pract. & Dig. Treat. 3:532

5. Popkin, R J (1956) The hydrogenated alkaloids of ergot (Hydergine) in geriatrics--Follow up study. Am. Pract. & Dig. Treat. 7:1594-1597.

6. Labecki, T D, Busby, C L (1954) Dihydrogenated ergot derivatives in cerebral arteriosclerosis. J. Geront. 9:485-486.

7. Hollister, L E (1955) Combined hydrogenated alkaloids of ergot in mental and nervous disorders associated with old age. Dis. Nerv. Syst. 26:1-4.

8. Forster, W, Schultz, S, Henderson, A L (1955) Combined hydrogenated alkaloids of ergot in senile and arteriosclerotic psychoses. Geriatrics 10(1):26-30.

9. Orma, E J (1956) Hydrogenated ergotalkaloids (Hydergine) in the treatment of geriatric postural dizziness. Ann. Med. Int. Fenn. 45:39-44.

10. Hofstatter, L, Ossoria, A, Mandl, B, Kohler, L H, Busch, A K, Hyman, A. (1956) Pharmaceutical treatment of patients with senile brain changes. Arch. Neurol. Psychiatr. (Chicago) 75:316-322.

11. Kaiser, G, Tschabitscher, H (1956) Erfahrungen mit Hydergin in der behandlung zerebraler durchblutungs storungen im hoheren Alter. Weiner Klin. Wochenschr. 9:150-154.

12. Banen, D M (1972) An ergot preparation (Hydergine) for relief of symptoms of cerebrovascular insufficiency. J. Am. Geriatr. Soc. 20:22-24.

13. Gerin, J (1969) Symptomatic treatment of cerebrovascular insufficiency with Hydergine. Curr. Ther. Res. 11:539-546.

14. Ditch, M, Kelly, F J, Resnick, O (1971) An ergot preparation in the treatment of cerebrovascular disorders in the geriatric patient: Double-blind study. J. Amer. Geriat. Soc. 19:208-217.

15. Jennings, W G (1972) An ergot alkaloid preparation (Hydergine) vs placebo for treatment of symptoms of cerebrovascular insufficiency: A double-blind study. J. Am. Geriatr. Soc. 10:407-412.

16. Rao, D B, Norris, J R (1972) A double-blind investigation of Hydergine in the treatment of cerebrovascular insufficiency in the elderly. Johns Hopkins Med. J. 130:317-324.

17. Triboletti, F, Ferri, H (1969) Hydergine for treatment of symptoms of cerebrovascular insufficiency. Curr. Ther. Res. 11:609-620.

18. Roubicek, J, Geiger, C H, Abt, K (1972) An ergot alkaloid preparation in geriatric therapy. J. Amer. Geriat. Soc. 20:222-229.

19. Thibault, A (1974) A double-blind evaluation of Hydergine and placebo in the treatment of patients with organic brain syndrome and cerebral arteriosclerosis in the nursing home. Curr. Med. Res. Opin. 2:482-487.

20. Novo, F P, Ryan, R P, Frazier, E L (1978) Dihydroergotoxine mesylate in treatment of symptoms of idiopathic cerebral dysfunction in geriatric patients. Clin. Ther. 1:359-369.

21. Gaitz, C M, Varner, R V, Overall, J E (1977) Pharmacotherapy for organic brain syndrome in late life. Arch. Gen. Psychiat. 34:839-845.

22. Rosen, H J (1975) Mental decline in the elderly: Pharmacotherapy (ergot alkaloids vs papaverine). J. Amer. Geriat. Soc. 23:169-174.

23. Bazo, A J (1973) An ergot alkaloid preparation (Hydergine) versus Papa-varine in treating common complaints of the aged: Double-blind study. J. Amer. Geriat. Soc. 21:63-71.

24. Nelson, J J (1975) Relieving select symptoms of the elderly. Geriatrics 30(3):133-142.

25. Yesavage, J A, Tinkleberg, J R, Hollister, L E, Berger, P A (1979) Vasodilators in senile dementias: A review of the literature. Arch. Gen. Psychiat. 36:220-223.

26. Emmenegger, H, Meier-Ruge, W (1968) The actions of Hydergine on the brain: A histochemical, circulatory and neurophysiological study. Pharmacology (Basel) 1:65-78.

27. Meier-Ruge, W, Iwangoff, P (1976) Biochemical effects of ergot alkaloids with special reference to the brain. Postgrad. Med. J. 52(Suppl. 1):47-54.

28. Tomlinson, B E, Blessed, G, Roth, M (1970) Observations on the brains of demented old people. J. Neurol. Sci. 11:205-242.

29. Salzmann, C, Kochansky, G E, Shader, R I (1972) Rating scales for geriatric psychopharmacology: A review. Psychopharm. Bull. 8:3-50.

30. Salzman, C, Shader, R I, Kochansky, G E (1972) Rating scales for psycho-tropic drug research with geriatric patients. (I) Behavior ratings. J. Amer. Geriat. Soc. 20:209-214

31. Salzman, C, Kochansky, G E, Shader, R I (1972) Rating scales for psycho-tropic drug research with geriatric patients. (II) Mood ratings. J. Amer. Geriat. Soc. 20:215-221.

32. Fanchamps, A (1978) Controlled studies of the effect of dihydroergo-toxine on the symptoms of senile cerebral insufficiency. Data on file at Sandoz, Inc., East Hanover, N.J.

33. Shader, R I, Harmatz, J S, Salzman, C (1974) A new scale for clinical assessment in geriatric populations: Sandoz Clinical Assessment--Geriatric (SCAG). J. Am. Geriat. Soc. 22:107-113.

34. Medical Letter (1977) Deapril-ST for senile dementia. Med. Letter on Drugs & Therapeutics 19:461-462.

35. Soni, S D, Soni, S S (1975) Dihydrogenated alkaloids of ergotoxine in non-hospitalized elderly patients. Curr. Med. Res. Op. 3:464-468.

36. Hollister, L E (1977) Mental disorders in the elderly. Drug Ther. 7:128-135.

37. Sathanathan, G L, Ferris, S, Gershon, S (1977) Aging: Current trends. In W. B. Essman and L. Valvelli (eds) Curr. Dev. in Psychopharmacology 4:251-264. NY:Spectrum Publ.

38. Cayley, A C, MacPherson, A, Wedgwood, J (1975) Sinus bradycardia following treatment with Hydergine for cerebrovascular insufficiency. Brit. Med. J. 2:384-385.

39. Kapoor, O P (1976) Iatrogenic ergot vasospastic angitis: A case report. Vasc. Surg. 10:58-60.

40. Physicians' Desk Referrence, Third edition (1979) p.1505. Oradell,NJ: Medical Economics.

CHOLINERGIC AGENTS IN SENILE DEMENTIA

JONATHAN O. COLE
Chief, Psychopharmacology Unit, McLean Hospital, 115 Mill Street, Belmont, Mass.
Consultant, Boston State Hospital, 591 Morton Street, Boston, Mass.

There is currently preliminary evidence suggesting that acetylcholine may have a role in memory and senile dementia. Choline acetyl transferase (CAT) is reduced in the brains of patients with senile dementia, making a resulting decrease in cholinergic activity probable as one aspect of the condition. This has been confirmed in 3 published studies on the levels of CAT in the brain of patients with senile dementia. Bowen et al, in the most detailed and rigorous available study, finds a 50% decrease in CAT levels in the parietal cortex of senile dementia patients as compared with aged normal controls.[1] Davies and Maloney find a concomitant fall in acetylcholinesterase activity which suggests, but by no means proves, the loss of cholinergic neurones[2] while Perry et al find a normal level of muscarinic receptors, suggesting that the post-synaptic cholinoceptive cells are intact.[3] In addition, McGeer and McGeer find a 70% decrease in CAT in a heterogeneous group of elderly brains as compared to brains from controls aged 20 - 50.[4] This study did not exclude brains from patients with dementia.

Thus, normal aging appears to be accompanied by a substantial decrease in CAT, while senile dementia is associated with a further reduction.

Increasing brain acetylcholine is of theoretical interest in a number of psychiatric and neurological conditions including tardive dyskinesia, Huntington's chorea, and mania as well as senile or presenile dementia. In the first three conditions, the abnormal state is believed to be due to dopaminergic overactivity (absolute or relative) in the brain; raising brain acetylcholine might improve the condition by correcting the balance between cholinergic and dopaminergic systems in the brain. In Huntington's disease there is also evidence that some, but not all, patients show a decrease in CAT in the basal ganglia.[5] Although large numbers of patients have not been treated with either choline or lecithin for any of the above conditions, a double-blind study has shown choline at about 10 grams a day to be more effective than placebo in reducing dyskinetic movements in chronic psychotic inpatients[6] and a few other cases of tardive dyskinesia, Huntington's chorea and mania have also been reported to improve on choline.[7] More recently, Growdon's group has used lecithin (about 1/5 phospha-tidylcholine) in a few cases of tardive dyskinesia with good results at doses up to 100 grams for about 3 months. Lecithin appears to be free of choline's tendency to make patients smell like dead fish and may have fewer gastro-intestinal cholinergic side effects as well.

Since both lecithin and choline have been shown to raise brain acetylcholine levels in experimental animals, it seems reasonable to assume that lecithin is the more acceptable agent for use in man. It should be noted that the Palo Alto group (K. Davis and P. Berger) feel strongly that choline, as the only available pure substance, deserves priority in studies because results obtained should be more clearly interpretable.[8] If lecithin is shown to be effective, there is always the possibility that its content of essential fatty acids or any of a large number of other constituents might be producing any observed effect.

To date, we are aware of only 3 studies of choline in senile dementia and 2 of lecithin, 1 unpublished, in presenile dementia.

Smith et al in London did a crossover study (2 weeks of choline bitartrate, 9 grams a day, 1 week washout, 2 weeks placebo) in 10 patients with senile dementia (mean age 77).[9] Three patients seemed less confused after 2 weeks on choline while 3 others showed increased urinary incontinence. Gastro-intestinal discomfort occurred in some patients. No statistically significant

changes were seen in a battery of cognitive and memory tests, perhaps because
of the short duration of study treatment.

Boyd et al from Edinburgh treated 7 elderly patients with choline (5 grams
a day for 2 weeks, then 10 grams a day for 2 weeks).[10] Again clinical observers
believed the patients became less irritable and more aware of their surroundings,
but the cognitive and behavioral measures used did not detect any clear changes.
The higher dose caused nausea and diarrhea. Two patients were improved on
testing, particularly in the first 24 hours of the trial.

Signoret et al treated 8 patients with Alzheimer's disease (ages 59 - 78)
with choline citrate (9 grams a day for 21 days).[11] The presentation of the
results defies understanding but apparently a few "younger" patients with shorter
duration of illness showed some improvement on memory tests as did some relatives
of patients who seem also to have been given choline.

Etienne et al treated 7 outpatients with Alzheimer's disease of less than 3
years duration with lecithin (Centrolex-F 3.7 grams choline per 100 grams
lecithin) in doses begining with 25 grams a day, increasing by 25 grams every
week for 4 weeks.[12] Plasma choline levels were increased from about 11 nmol./
ml. to 38 nmol./ml. Three patients showed some improvement on paired associate
learning and 2 of these showed improved visual retention. No changes occurred
on immediate or remote memory or constructional ability. Some digestive side
effects were noted, but no foul odor, depression or cholinergic toxicity.
The average tolerated lecithin dose was around 75 grams a day.

At a recent meeting, Christie reported on the use of lecithin (20-30%
phosphatidylcholine) at 100 grams a day in 11 patients with presenile dementia
(average age 60, average duration 3.8 years).[13] Patients received choline up
to 5 grams a day for 5 days before going on to lecithin. The 1 least impaired
and the 7 most impaired patients showed no change, but the 3 intermediate
patients improved on lecithin in orientation, speech and dyspraxia. One

patient became more irritable on choline and in general choline slightly wors-
ened ward behavior while lecithin slightly improved ward behavior. One patient
has now been maintained on lecithin for a year with no further deterioration.

In general, the available studies suffer from small sample size and short
durations of treatment. They show suggestive changes. Some patients with
senile or presenile dementia may respond to choline or lecithin with mild
degrees of improvement which may be more apparent in general social functioning
than on discrete memory tasks, though both may improve. Lecithin seems reasonably well tolerated though higher dosages may cause anorexia and gastrointestinal discomfort. The foul odor caused by choline does not seem to occur.
Depression, which has been reported to occur occasionally with choline use in
tardive dyskinesia,[14] has not been reported in senile dementia patients on
lecithin or choline to date.

There is some evidence also that cholinergic drugs may improve memory
generally. There is 1 study of a single patient with a memory defect caused
by herpes simplex encephalitis who was given several doses of physostigmine
in a double-blind trial.[15] An "impressive" gain on a selective reminding
memory test was observed on 0.8 mg of physostigmine given subscutaneously,
but not after higher or lower dosages. The authors felt the data suggested a
drug effect on both memory storage and retrieval. The patient seemed calmer
and more goal directed during testing on the proper physostigmine dose.

Davis et al have studied the effects of a 1-hour intravenous infusion of
1.0 mgs of physostigmine on memory in normal volunteers, using a double-blind
crossover design with a saline placebo control.[16] Physostigmine had no effect
on short term memory and only a suggestive effect on retrieval of words learned
before drug administration. However, both learning and retrieval were improved
by physostigmine on a word list learned after half the drug had been given.

Sitaram et al studied the effects of arecoline (4 mg) and scopolamine (0.5

mgs) on trials to criterion in learning 10 words from a familiar category (e.g. vegetables).[17] Arecoline (with possible peripheral side effects blocked by methscopolamine 0.3 mg) improved learning and memory and scopolamine impaired it relative to placebo. Arecoline at 6 mgs i.m. reversed the effects of scopolamine on learning and memory. A single 10 gram oral dose of choline chloride was also compared to placebo in normal subjects on the ability to learn lists of 10 un-categorized words to criterion. Choline improved performance significantly. Subjects who performed less well on these learning tasks in either study showed significantly larger drug effects with all 3 drugs tested. Mohs et al report a similar trend in their physostigmine study.[18]

Drachman has observed that scopolamine (1 mg s.c.) interferes with ongoing memory storage and with retrieval of information from old memory in normal subjects and also produces a pattern of changes on the Wechsler Adult Intel-ligence Scale (impairment on performance scores) similar to that seen in senile dementia.[19] He mentions an uncontrolled pilot study of 0.8 of physo-stigmine s.c. in 13 normal aged subjects which showed a trend toward improved memory storage and performance. Other controlled studies of the effects of scopolamine in normal volunteers [89, 92] have shown impairment of the registra-tion and recall of new information; very short term tasks like digits forward are not impaired.

Thus, there are suggestions in the available literature that cholinergic drugs at a proper dose may improve retention and recall in both normal and organically impaired subjects on tasks where there is room for improvement. It may be possible to improve psychological functioning in the elderly with cholinergic agents even if the basic defect in senile dementia is not a loss of cholinergic function in the central nervous system. If the elderly in general and senile dementias in particular have a major loss in presynaptic cholinergic neurones, then drugs like choline and lecithin which require, presumably, conversion into acetylcholine intracellularly as well as drugs like physostigmine which block the destruction of synthesized acetylcholine should be more effective in patients showing lesser degrees of cholinergic cell loss. If, in more severe degrees of dementia, cholinergic neurones are lost but post-synaptic receptors are intact, arecoline (a direct cholinergic agonist) might be more effective. There is also a suggestion that dose may be a crucial issue; too low a dose should be ineffective while too high a dose might both cause cholinergic side effects and interfere with learning or memory.

REFERENCES

1. Bowen, D. et al (1976) Neurotransmitter-related enzymes and indices of hypoxia in senile dementia and other abiotrophies. Brain. 99 pp. 459-496.
2. Davies, P. et al (1976) Selective loss of central cholinergic neurones in Alzheimer's disease. Lancet. 2, pp. 1403.
3. Perry, E. et al (1977) Necropsy evidence of central cholinergic deficits in senile dementia. Lancet. 1, pp. 189.
4. McGeer, E. and McGeer, P. (1976) Neurotransmitter metabolism in the aging brain. In Terry, R. and Gershon, S. (Eds.) Neurobiology of Aging. Raven Press, New York. pp. 389-404.
5. Bird, E. (1978) The brain in Huntington's chorea. Psychol. Med. 8. pp. 357-360.
6. Growdon J. et al (1977) Oral choline administration to patients with tardive dyskinesia. New England J. of Med. 297. pp. 524-527.
7. Jenden, D. (1978) The neurochemical basis of acetylcholine precursor loading as a therapeutic strategy. In Davis, K and Berger, P. (Eds.) Brain Acetylcholine and Neuropsychiatric Disease. Plenum Press.
8. Davis, K. (1978) Clinical and preclinical experience with choline chloride in Huntington's disease and tardive dyskinesia. Paper presented at the Symposium on the Uses of Choline and Lecithin in Neurologic and Psychiatric Diseases, Tuscon, Arizona.
9. Smith, C. et al (1978) Choline therapy in Alzheimer's disease. Lancet. 2, pp. 318.
10. Boyd, W. et al (1977) Clinical effects of choline in Alzheimer senile dementia. Lancet. 2, pp. 711.
11. Signoret, J. et al (1978) Influence of choline on amnesia in early Alzheimer's disease. Lancet. 2, pp. 837.
12. Etienne, P. et al (1978) Lecithin in Alzheimer's disease. Lancet. 2, pp. 1206.
13. Christie, J. (1978) Effects of choline and lecithin administration to patients with Alzheimer's disease. Paper presented at Symposium on the Uses of Choline and Lecithin in Neurologic and Psychiatric Diseases. Tuscon, Arizona.

14. Tamminga, C. (1979) Choline and lecithin in affective illness. In Growdon, J., Wurtman, R. and Barbeau, A. (Eds.) Uses of Choline and Lecithin in Neurological and Psychiatric Disorders. Raven Press, New York.
15. Peters, B., Levin H. (1977) Memory enhancement after physostigmine treatment in the amnestic syndrom. Arch. of Neurol. 34, pp. 215-219.
16. Davis, K. et al (1978) Physostigmine: improvement of long-term memory processes in normal humans. Science. 201, pp. 272-274.
17. Sitaram, N. et al (1978) Human serial learning: enhancement with arecoline and choline and impairment with scopolamine. Science. 201, pp.274-276.
18. Mohs, et al (1977) Physostigmine in cholinergic aspects of human memory. Paper presented at the VI World Congress of Psychiatry. Honolulu.
19. Drachman, D. (1978) Central cholinergic system and memory. In Lipton, M., DiMascio, A. and Killam, K. (Eds) Psychopharmacology: A Generation of Progress. Raven Press, New York. pp.651-662.
20. Safer, D., Allen, R. (1971) The central effects of scopolamine in man. Biological Psychiat. 3, pp.347-355.

CLINICAL TRIALS OF GEROVITAL H3 IN THE TREATMENT OF DEPRESSION IN THE ELDERLY

WILLIAM W.K. ZUNG, M.D.   AND HSIOH-SHAN WANG, M.B.
Professor of Psychiatry, Duke University Medical Center, Durham, NC 27710

INTRODUCTION

Current interest and impetus in the area of aging has focused on several areas including the treatment of disorders associated with aging such as depressive disorders. In the area of psychopharmacology, the compound Gerovital H3 (GH3) and its principal component procaine hydrochloride have had reports of its therapeutic efficacy[1-2], as well as its swan song[3], in both the medical and lay press. In a field of scientific inquiry where the state-of-the-art has changed rapidly within the span of the numerous reports published, there appears to be more heat than light generated by both medical and lay writers of the controversy with regards to the role of GH3 or procaine hydrochloride in the armamentarium of the medical practitioner. Several scholarly and comprehensive reviews of the literature on GH3 and procaine compounds have been published, and the reader is directed towards them for their full and excellent texts[4,5].

Since the 1956 report by Aslan entitled: "A new method for prophylaxis and treatment of aging with Novocain: Eutropic and rejuvenating effects" appeared in Therapiewoche[1], there has been a great deal of interest in the drug GH3. GH3 is a solution containing 2% procaine hydrochloride with benzoic acid added as a preservative and potassium metabisulfite as an antioxidant. According to Aslan, GH3 is not plain procaine HCl, and the pharmacology of GH3 and procaine are not the same. The molecular structure of procaine consists of an aromatic ring connected through an intermediate chain with an amino group, an ester linkage being present in this intermediate chain. Procaine when injected in the human body is rapidly hydrolyzed by cholinesterase into para-aminobenzoic acid (PABA) and diethylaminoethanol (DEAE). In the case of procaine in the GH3 formula, metabolic studies using thin layer chromatography techniques show that the intact molecules of procaine can be found in blood and urine after six hours of the administration of the drug. She gives two possible explanations for this difference: 1. The acid pH of the solution produces a slow release mechanism for procaine, and 2. The benzoic acid forms a loose complex with procaine, protecting it against the action of cholinesterase. The issue of pharmacological differences between procaine in the formulation of the Romanian GH3 and plain procaine has not been resolved in vivo.

The purpose of this presentation is to summarize the results of studies that used GH3 as the investigational drug for its potential therapeutic effect in the treatment of depressive disorders, and more specifically in the elderly population.

OPEN TRIALS

Two open trials have been conducted using GH3, and separately reported. Sakalis, Gershon and Shopsin[6] treated 10 patients, ages 63-82, with diagnoses of senile-arteriosclerotic dementia with features of depression, with GH3 for three weeks. The dosage schedule was: 100 mg x 3 for the 1st week, 150 mg x 3 for the 2nd week, and 200 mg x 3 for the 3rd week, for a possible maximum dosage of 1,350 mg of procaine over the study period. Ratings for depression were made using the Clinical Global Impression for Improvement (CGI:I), Hamilton Rating scale for Depression (HRD), and the Nurses Observation Scale for Inpatient Evaluation (NOSIE). Results reported by them showed no significant change on the CGI, while two factors derived from the HRD were significantly improved (somatization factor, and anxiety/depression factor) with p values of 0.05, and 0.01, respectively. No side effects were noted, and the authors interpreted their results as GH3 having a mild euphoriant effect. Retrospectively, a comparison of the dosage and duration of treatment used in this study to dosages and duration used in later studies may account for their equivocal results.

Cohen and Ditman reported an open study using 17 normal volunteers with mild depression and fatigue as common complaints, 17 psychiatric patients with moderate to severe depressions, and 7 medical patients with concomitant depression with their chronic illnesses[7]. The age range of these subjects was from 40-85 years old. The dosage schedule of GH3 used was 100-200 mg, x 3 for 4 weeks, for a total of 12 injections. The maximum possible dosage equals 1,200 mg of procaine. Evaluations for depression were performed by using a psychiatric interview, a mood scale, and the Zung Self-rating Depression Scale. The authors reported that 85% of the 41 subjects showed some improvement, with the following breakdown: 15 of the 17 normal volunteers, 14 of the 17 psychiatric patients, and 6 of the 7 medical patients. Improvements were noted in: sense of well-being, increased energy, increased relaxation, better sleeping time, memory and thinking, and decreased physical discomfort. There were minimal side-effects reported. The authors noted that 9 patients with elevated serum cholesterol levels had lower levels post-treatment (mean pre-treatment = 339 mg% cholesterol, post-treatment = 289 mg%).

DOUBLE-BLIND TRIALS

Four double-blind studies using injectable GH3 versus placebo have been conducted. The first double-blind study was performed by Zung, Gianturco, Pfeiffer, Wang, Whanger, Bridge, and Potkin comparing injectable GH3 versus oral imipramine, using appropriate injectable and oral placebos[8]. The other three double-blind studies used identical protocols investigating the therapeutic efficacy of GH3 versus placebo, and were performed by Kurland and Hayman[9], Jarvik and Olsen[10], and Cammer[11]. Table 1 summarizes the number of subjects studied, age, and mean total GH3 dosage, in mg of procaine hydrochloride used in the studies.

TABLE 1. CLINICAL TRIALS OF GH3 IN FOUR STUDIES

INVESTIGATOR		GH3	PBO	IMI
Zung et al	N=	9	10	11
	Age, mean	67.2	68.7	68.5
	Age, range	61-77	63-74	60-79
	GH3, mean			
	total dosage	2,022 mg		
Kurland and Hayman	N =	33	30	
	Age, mean	59.2	58.9	
	Age, range	45-84	45-83	
	GH3, mean			
	total dosage	2,100 mg		
Jarvik and Olsen	N =	11	13	
	Age, mean	59.1	60.1	
	Age, range	48-77	48-78	
	GH3, mean			
	total dosage	2,100 mg		
Cammer	N =	20	20	
	Age, mean	60.0	60.4	
	Age, range	51-70	50-74	
	GH3, mean			
	total dosage	2,110 mg		

Data from the first three double-blind studies have been combined, and a single set of statistical analyses are presented. The common goal of each study is that of investigating the possible therapeutic efficacy of GH3 in the treatment of depressive disorders as they occur in the elderly, in a double-blind study comparing GH3 versus placebo. The test preparations used were as follows: 1. GH3 was supplied in 5 cc ampules each containing 100 mg

of 2% procaine hydrochlorida manufactured in Romania. 2. Placebo in the form
of normal saline in matching ampules.

Patient Selection. Suitable for consideration for the studies were outpatients 45 years old and over, with no upper limit as to age, no restrictions
as to sex, who had depressive disorders of at least mild in global severity.
This was determined by using a Clinical Global Impression (CGI) scale of 1 to
7, with 3 = mildly ill. In the studies, a depressive disorder was operation-
ally defined as manifesting: 1. A mood disturbance which is characterized by
pervasive feelings and complaints of being depressed, sad, and tearful. 2.
Physiological symptoms which include diurnal variation, disturbances of sleep,
decreased appetite, decreased weight, decreased libido, constipation, tachy-
cardia, and unexplainable fatigue. 3. Psychomotor disturbances which are
either that of retardation or agitation. 4. Psychological disturbances which
include confusion, emptiness, hopelessness, indecisiveness, irritability, dis-
satisfaction, personal devaluation, and suicidal rumination.

The following patients were excluded from the study: 1. Actively suicidal
patients. 2. Patients who were incapable of spontaneous conversation and
activity. 3. Patients who were severely demented. 4. Patients who were
schizophrenic, or had evidences of a thought disorder. 5. Patients who were
on the following medications: sulfonamides, neostigmine or physostigmine.
Lastly, patients were to have been free of all psychotropic drugs for at least
seven days prior to entry to the study protocol.

Study Design

All patients were skin tested for potential sensitivity to known GH3 prior
to the administration of test preparations, and the results of the skin testing read immediately and after 24 hours (negative in all cases).

These were all double-blind studies of 4 weeks in duration. All patients
received i.m. medication using the following schedule: Week 1 - 5 cc, 3 times
a week. Weeks 2, 3 and 4 - 10 cc (two 5 cc ampules), 3 times a week. This
is equivalent to a total dosage of 2,100 mg of procaine hydrochloride.

The Zung et al study was performed by comparing GH3 versus placebo versus
imipramine. For the purpose of this combined data analysis, the patients who
received imipramine have been omitted.

Evaluation Procedures

The common behavioral measurements made across the three studies to be reported here were: 1. Clinical Global Impression for severity of illness

(CGI:S), 2. Clinical Global Impression for improvement of illness (CGI:I),
3. Hamilton Rating scale for Depression (HRD), which was used in two of the
three studies, and 4. Zung Self-rating Depression Scale (SDS). These measures
were made pre-treatment and post-treatment, with mid-treatment measures made for
CGI:I.

Results

Combining results from the three separate studies, a total of 53 patients
received GH3, and a total of 53 patients received placebo (PBO).

The combined results and data analyses for the depression measurements made
are summarized in Tables 2-7.

TABLE 2. T-tests comparing pre- and post-treatment variables measured of patients treated with Gerovital H3.

TX=GH3	PRE-TX M (s.d.)	POST-TX M (s.d.)	P
CGI:S	4.2 (1.0)	2.5 (1.4)	.01
HRD	48.0 (20.9)	29.6 (16.9)	.01
SDS	59.6 (13.8)	47.1 (13.1)	.01
	MID-TX	POST-tx	P
CGI:I	2.9 (1.3)	2.2 (1.2)	.01

TABLE 3. T-tests comparing pre- and post-treatment variables measured of patients treated with placebo.

TX=PBO	PRE-TX M (s.d.)	POST-TX M (s.d.)	P
CGI:S	4.1 (0.9)	3.6 (1.2)	.01
HRD	44.7 (19.6)	39.6 (20.4)	.01
SDS	61.9 (10.6)	56.3 (13.4)	.01
	MID-TX	POST-TX	P
CGI:I	3.5 (1.0)	3.5 (1.4)	n.s.

TABLE 4. T-tests comparing Clinical Global Impression for severity of illness. Analysis of covariance (ANOCOVA) performed by using pre-treatment scores as the covariate.

TX GROUP	CGI:S PRE-TX M (s.d.)	P
GH3	4.2 (1.0)	n.s.
PBO	4.1 (0.9)	
	CGI:S POST-TX	
GH3	2.5 (1.4)	.01
PBO	3.6 (1.2)	
	ANOCOVA	.01
	CGI:S CHANGE SCORE	
GH3	1.7 (1.3)	.01
PBO	0.5 (1.0)	

TABLE 5. T-tests comparing Clinical Global Impression for improvement of illness. Analysis of covariance (ANOCOVA) performed by using mid-treatment scores as the covariate.

TX GROUP	CGI:I MID-TX M (s.d.)	P
GH3	2.9 (1.3)	.02
PBO	3.5 (1.0)	
	CGI:I POST-TX	
GH3	2.2 (1.2)	.01
PBO	3.5 (1.4)	
	ANOCOVA	.01
	CGI:I CHANGE SCORE	
GH3	0.7 (1.2)	.02
PBO	0.0 (1.3)	

Statistical analyses comparing pre-treatment with post-treatment results of scores obtained on the CGI:S, HRD and SDS showed significant improvement at the end of the 28-day treatment period on all measures. (All p values are two-tailed, and have been corrected for multiple t-tests to protect against spurious statistical significances.) In addition, on comparing CGI for improvement of illness, which were measured at mid-treatment and post-treatment, the GH3 treated patients improved significantly between these two time intervals (see Table 2).

Table 3 summarizes the within group data for all patients treated with placebo. Statistical analyses comparing pre- with post-treatment results of scores obtained on the CGI:S, HRD and SDS showed significant improvement at the end of the 28-day period on all measures. Comparing CGI for improvement of illness, which were measured at mid- and post-treatment, placebo patients did not improve between these two time intervals.

Table 4 summarizes the between group data comparison on the behavioral measure of CGI:S, at pre- and post-treatment, and as a change score. The change score is derived by subtracting the post-treatment score from the pre-treatment score for each patient. We can see that the two treatment groups started out at the same level of psychopathology as measured by the CGI:S (p=n.s.), but the GH3 patients improved significantly better than did the PBO patients as evidenced by the post-treatment, and by the change score results, with both p's = 0.01. An analysis of covariance (ANOCOVA) was performed on all data generated from these studies. The ANOCOVA was performed in all instances by using the pre-treatment scores as the covariate. Results of the ANOCOVA between GH3 and placebo treated patients show that the GH3 group improved at a statistically significant level.

Table 5 compares the CGI:I results. The improvement as rated by the CGI:I at mid-treatment is significantly different, with the GH3 group showing more improvement. These improvement differences were still significantly different at post-treatment, with the GH3 treated group showing greater improvement than the PBO group.

Table 6 compares the HRD results. The two groups started at the same level of psychopathology at pre-treatment (p=n.s.), but the GH3 group improved more (significantly lower HRD scores) as evidenced by the post-treatment, change score and ANOCOVA results.

Table 7 summarizes the SDS results. Statistical analyses comparing GH3 and PBO treated patients at pre-treatment showed that the two groups started at the same level of psychopathology (p=n.s.) as measured by the SDS. After treatment, the GH3 patients improved more at post-treatment, by change scores, and the ANOCOVA results.

TABLE 6. T-tests comparing Hamilton Rating Scale for Depression (HRD) between the two treatment groups. Analysis of covariance (ANOCOVA) performed by using pre-treatment scores as the covariate.

TX GROUP	HRD PRE-TX M	(s.d.)	P
GH3	48.0	(20.9)	n.s.
PBO	44.7	(19.6)	

	HRD POST-TX		
GH3	29.6	(16.9)	.02
PBO	39.6	(20.4)	

	ANOCOVA		.01

	HRD CHANGE SCORE		
GH3	18.5	(12.3)	.01
PBO	5.1	(9.1)	

TABLE 7. T-tests comparing Zung Self-rating Depression Scale between the two treatment groups. Analysis of covariance (ANOCOVA) performed by using pre-treatment scores as the covariate.

TX GROUP	SDS PRE-TX M	(s.d.)	P
GH3	59.6	(13.8)	n.s.
PBO	61.9	(10.6)	

	SDS POST-TX		
GH3	47.1	(13.1)	.01
PBO	56.3	(13.4)	

	ANOCOVA		.01

	SDS CHANGE SCORE		
GH3	12.4	(14.3)	.01
PBO	5.5	(11.2)	

Cammer's study used the identical above described patient selection criteria, as well as identical study design and dosage schedule.

The following evaluations were performed pre-treatment on Day 0, and repeated on Day 14 and on post-treatment whch was Day 28:

1. Clinical Global Impression for Severity of Illness (CGI:S)

2. Zung Depression Status Inventory (DSI)

3. Zung Self-rating Depression Scale (SDS)

4. Katz Adjustment Scale for Socially-Expected Activities (KAS S-EA)

5. Katz Adjustment Scale for Free-time Activities (KAS F-TA)

On Days 14 and 28, a Clinical Global Impression for Improvement of Illness (CGI:I) was entered.

Results of his study for within-treatment group, using 2-tailed, paired t-tests are summarized in Tables 8 and 9.

TABLE 8. T-tests comparing pre-treatment with post-treatment variables
measured (Clinical Global Impression:Severity of Illness, Depression
Status Inventory, Self-rating Depression Scale, Katz Adjustment Scale
for Socially-Expected Activities, and for Free-time Activities, Clinical
Global Impression:Improvement of illness) obtained from patients treated
with Gerovital H3 (N=20)

VARIABLE	Pre-treatment m	(s.d.)	Post-treatment m	(s.d.)	P
CGI:S	3.2	(0.4)	1.6	(0.7)	<.05
DSI	61.7	(4.1)	37.9	(7.8)	<.05
SDS	63.5	(7.7)	47.3	(12.7)	<.05
KAS S-E A	28.2	(4.8)	30.2	(5.0)	n.s.
KAS F-T A	42.2	(9.3)	39.8	(7.4)	n.s.

	Mid-treatment m	(s.d.)	Post-treatment m	(s.d.)	P
CGI:I	2.6	(0.5)	1.9	(1.0)	<.05

TABLE 9. T-tests comparing pre-treatment with post-treatment variables
measured (Clinical Global Impression:Severity of Illness, Depression
Status Inventory, Self-rating Depression Scale, Katz Adjustment Scale
for Socially-Expected Activities, and for Free-time Activities, Clinical
Global Impression:Improvement of illness) obtained from patients treated
with placebo (N=20).

VARIABLE	Pre-treatment m	(s.d.)	Post-treatment m	(s.d.)	P
CGI:S	3.2	(0.4)	3.1	(0.2)	n.s.
DSI	61.0	(6.0)	58.7	(6.0)	n.s.
SDS	66.0	(8.1)	63.1	(7.3)	n.s.
KAS S-E A	28.0	(5.6)	25.5	(5.6)	<.05
KAS F-T A	44.1	(8.0)	40.9	(7.8)	n.s.

	Mid-treatment m	(s.d.)	Post-treatment m	(s.d.)	P
CGI:I	3.7	(0.6)	3.7	(0.6)	n.s.

Patients treated with GH3 improved significantly on the CGI for severity of
illness, and for improvement of illness, Zung DSI, and Zung SDS indices (p =
less than 0.05 in all instances), while changes on the KAS scales were not
significant. Patients treated with placebo did not improve, and there were
no statistically significant differences between pre- and post-treatment scores
on the CGI:S, CGI:I, Zung DSI, or Zung SDS indices. The KAS socially-expected
activity scale showed a significant decrease over time, denoting that the
placebo-treated patients had a decrease in their activities.

During the clinical trial no patient-reported side effects occurred in the placebo-treated group. In the GH3 treated group, the only reported side effect thought to be drug attributable was that of dizziness. This occurred in three patients, each of whom had a single episode of feeling mildly dizzy. The symptom disappeared with rest.

Summary of the Four Double-blind Studies

Evidence for the therapeutic efficacy of GH3 as an antidepressant was demonstrated on all of the behavioral measurements studied. These included: Clinical Global Impression for Severity of illness, Clinical Global Impression for Improvement of illness, Hamilton Rating scale for Depression, Zung Depression Status Inventory, and the Zung Self-rating Depression Scale. Statistical analyses (using analysis of variance and analysis of covariance) of data obtained on these ratings performed between treatment groups showed that the GH3 treated patients improved significantly more than did the placebo treated patients at post-treatment, as well as on change scores (pre-treatment value minus post-treatment value).

Special Studies and Analyses

1. Cholesterol levels

A previous report on the results of an open trial of GH3 indicated that this drug may lower serum cholesterol levels[7]. In order to test this possibility, we selected for further data analysis, all patients from the Zung, Kurland, and Jarvik studies who had serum cholesterol levels of 250 mg% or above at pre-treatment, and compared their cholesterol levels at post-treatment, by the two treatment groups. Results of this data analysis are found in Table 10.

TABLE 10. T-tests comparing pre-treatment with post-treatment cholesterol levels of GH3 and placebo-treated patients whose pre-treatment cholesterol levels were 250 mg % and above.

TX	N	m (s.d.) CHOLESTEROL, mg % PRE-TREATMENT		m (s.d.) CHOLESTEROL, mg % POST-TREATMENT		P
GH3	19	293.8	(42.6)	278.1	(31.0)	.05
PBO	13	270.6	(18.5)	281.6	(36.9)	n.s.

We can see that there were 19 GH3 treated patients who had serum cholesterol levels of 250 mg or above at pre-treatment. At post-treatment, the mean cholesterol values for this group of patients decreased, and at a significant level. There were 13 placebo treated patients who had at pre-treatment

cholesterol levels of 250 mg or above. At post-treatment, the mean cholesterol
levels for this population of patients showed an increase, which was not statistically significant.

2. Cognitive function

Patients with depressive disorders have been found to have cognitive impairment which is measureable with psychometric testing, and such deficits in
cognitive functioning in depressed patients improve with treatment with antidepressant drugs[12]. In addition, depression in the elderly patient may be
present in the setting of cognitive impairment secondary to aging, and/or an
organic brain syndrome. In order to document the status of cognitive functioning of the patients in our study, as well as study the effects of treatment on
cognitive functioning, all patients were tested using the Wechsler Memory Scale
(WMS). During the pre-treatment period, WMS form I was used, and during the
post-treatment period, WMS form II was used. Results of the study are in
Table 11.

TABLE 11. Comparison of the Wechsler Memory Scale Mental
Quotient results obtained from the three treatment groups
tested pre-, and post-treatment with GH3, imipramine, or
placebo.

TX GROUP	TEST PERIOD	WMS MQ m (s.d.)	WMS MQ CHANGE SCORE m (s.d.)
GH3	Pre-tx	94.0 (21.1)	2.6 (10.5)
	Post-tx	96.6 (24.4)	
IMI	Pre-tx	103.6 (20.7)	8.0 (12.3)
	Post-tx	111.6 (17.5)	
PBO	Pre-tx	100.1 (13.3)	10.1 (9.9)
	Post-tx	110.2 (10.0)	

Statistical analyses using ANOVA showed that the pre-treatment WMS MQ scores
were not significantly different from each other among the three treatment
groups, nor were the post-treatment scores, nor were the change scores (calculated by subtracting the pre-treatment and post-treatment scores) significantly
different from each other. Thus, the WMS MQ documented the cognitive status of
the patients in the study as being within the normal range. While the change
scores were not statistically significant, all three treatment groups showed an
increase in their MQ scores.

3. Cerebral functioning and neurophysiological effects

Aging is associated with many physiological and pathological changes

involving the cardiovascular, pulmonary, the CNS and many other systems. The
brain is known to undergo considerable loss of neurons and degenerative changes
in old age. The cerebral arteries of older people are also most likely affected
by atherosclerotic changes of varying degrees. In patients with significant
cerebral atherosclerosis, cerebral vascular resistance is increased and the
auto-regulatory mechanism in the cerebral vascular system is impaired. The
auto-regulatory mechanism, when intact, makes the cerebral blood flow independent of the systemic blood pressure. When this mechanism is impaired, the cerebral blood flow becomes more dependent on the blood pressure and more vulnerable
to the change of blood pressure. A fall in blood pressure, which would hardly
be noticeable to persons with normal vessels, may significantly affect the cerebral hemodynamics in persons with cerebral atherosclerosis.

Because of these changes, many elderly patients cannot tolerate certain drugs
that have clearly been proven for their therapeutic efficacy and safety in
younger adult patients. For example, tricyclic antidepressants have long been
the drug of choice for depression. Nevertheless, these drugs have a marked
anticholinergic effect which may cause or aggravate many disorders commonly
associated with aging, such as urinary retention, constipation, glaucoma, and
cardiac arrhythmias. This anticholinergic effect probably also plays an important role in the development of acute confusional state often seen in elderly patients receiving these drugs. Postural hypotension is another common
side effect of tricyclic antidepressants. This may lead to symptoms and signs
attributable to a diffuse or localized ischemic disorder of the brain.

In investigating the new drug used primarily in the aged, the adverse effect
is as important as, or at times even more important than, the efficacy in a
given use. We were interested to study the comparative effects of GH3 on the
brain with those of imipramine and placebo. Electroencephalograph (EEG) was
used to evaluate the effect on electrocortical activities of the brain and the
Xenon-133 inhalation method was used to evaluate the cerebral blood flow.

All EEG's were recorded with an 8-channel Grass Electroencephalograph, using
both monopolar and bipolar techniques. From each record, samples of the occipital rhythm, totaling 20 seconds, were measured manually. The average frequency
per second was the occipital dominant frequency.

Cerebral blood flow was determined by the Xenon-133, inhalation method described by Obrist and his co-workers[13].

Results

Table 12 summarizes the CBF and EEG findings. Both pre-treatment and post-treatment CBF and EEG frequency were not significantly different among these three groups. The difference between the two repeated measurements was not significant within each group or between groups. The imipramine group, nevertheless, appeared to show a relatively greater post-treatment decrease in CBF and EEG frequency as compared with placebo and GH3 groups.

Table 12 also summarizes the mean arterial blood pressure (MABP) which is the sum of one-third of the pulse pressure and diastolic blood pressure. The only statistical significance was the post-treatment decline of MABP in the imipramine group (from 102 mm. Hg. to 89.5 mm. Hg.) at the .05 level.

TABLE 12. Comparison of the cerebral blood flow, EEG, and arterial BP data for the three treatment groups at pre-treatment, post-treatment, and difference scores ($\overline{d}$). *P = 0.05 level of significance.

	Average Cerebral Blood Flow (ml/100 gm/min)			EEG Occipital Frequency (Hz)			Mean Arterial BP (mm Hg)		
	Pre-tx	Post-tx	$\overline{d}$	Pre-tx	Post-tx	$\overline{d}$	Pre-tx	Post-tx	$\overline{d}$
GEROVITAL H3									
Mean	55.0	54.6	-0.4	9.19	9.01	-0.17	96.2	90.8	-5.4
S.D.	10.7	10.7	9.6	1.42	1.40	1.02	11.9	11.6	10.6
IMIPRAMINE									
Mean	53.7	49.8	-3.9	9.64	9.02	-0.62	102.1	89.5	-12.6*
S.D.	13.4	11.5	8.9	1.30	1.35	1.33	12.7	15.4	14.0
PLACEBO									
Mean	47.3	47.0	-0.3	9.03	9.27	0.24	98.2	94.2	- 4.0
S.D.	5.5	8.3	6.4	1.03	0.87	0.85	10.7	13.5	13.4

Discussion

Because the number of patients in our study was relatively small and many variables were involved, one should be cautious in drawing any definite conclusion from the findings presented; nevertheless, several points warrant emphasizing. Perusal of individual data show: First, five patients showed a significant change of CBF (increase or decrease of more than 18%) which was most likely related to the changes of blood pressure. The relationship between CBF changes and blood pressure changes, in general, follows two patterns that have long been recognized. (1) Abnormally high blood pressure is associated with a reduction of CBF. When the high blood pressure is corrected, the CBF improves. It most likely occurs in elderly patients having so-called essential hypertension and probably little cerebral artherosclerosis. (2) In some elderly, a relatively high blood pressure is needed to maintain an adequate blood supply to the brain and a small drop in blood pressure, though still within normal range, may result in a significant reduction of CBF. This most likely occurs in the elderly persons having moderate to severe cerebral artherosclerosis.

Since the individual variations are rather great and cannot be accurately predicted, one must be very cautious in using drugs that may lower the blood pressure in the aged group.

In the 10 patients treated with imipramine, two showed a significant reduction of CBF which was related to a drop of blood pressure and two others showed a marked slowing of EEG frequency. The slowing of EEG frequency has also been observed by others on patients receiving imipramine. Nevertheless, the underlying mechanism of such a slowing associated with imipramine is still unclear. Slowing of EEG frequency is usually a common finding in many metabolic, toxic or circulatory disorders of the brain. In our study, severe confusional state was observed in one, but not the other patient who showed such a marked slowing of EEG frequency. In the GH3 group, no significant reduction of CBF or marked slowing of EEG frequency was observed. This may suggest that for elderly patients, GH3 can be considered as a safer drug than imipramine as far as the adverse effects on the brain is concerned.

ACKNOWLEDGEMENT

Dr. Alfred Sapse of Rom-Amer Pharmaceuticals made the data available on the double-blind studies which was used in this report.

REFERENCES

1. Aslan, A. (1956) A new method for the prophylaxis and treatment of aging with Novocain: Eutropic and rejuvenating effects. Die Therapiewoche, 7, 14.

2. Aslan, A. (1974) Theoretical and practical aspects of chemotherapeutic techniques in the retardation of the aging process, in Theoretical Aspects of Aging, M. Rockstein, M.L. Sussman, and J. Chesky, eds, Academic Press, New York.

246

3. New Drugs and Developments in Therapeutics: Procaine - Its Song is Ended, Editorial (1962), Council on Drugs, J.A.M.A., 180, 965.

4. Jarvik, L.F. and Milne, J.E. (1975) Gerovital-H3: A Review of the Literature, In: Aging, Vol. 2, Gershon, A. and Raskin, A., eds, Raven Press, New York.

5. Ostfeld, A., Smith, C.M. and Stotsky, B.A. (1977) The Systemic Use of Procaine in the Treatment of the Elderly: A Review, J. Am. Geriatrics Soc. 25, 1-19.

6. Sakalis, G., Gershon, S. and Shopsin, B. (1974) A trial of Gerovital H3 in Depression During Senility, Curr. Therap. Res., 16, 59-63.

7. Cohen, S. and Ditman, K.S. (1974) Gerovital H3 in the Treatment of the Depressed Aging Patient, Psychosom. 14, 15.

8. Zung, W.W.K., Gianturco, D., Pfeiffer, E., Wang, H.S., Whanger, A., Bridge, P. and Potkin, S. (1974) Pharmacology of Depression in the Aged: Evaluation of Gerovital H3 as an Antidepressans Drug, Psychosom. 15, 127-131.

9. Kurland, M.L. and Hayman, M. (1976) A Procaine Derivative for the Treatment of Depression in an Outpatient Population, Psychosom. 17, 96-102.

10. Jarvik, L. and Olsen (1975) A double-blind Study of Gerovital H3 in the Treatment of Depression.

11. Cammer, L. (1975) Gerovital H3 Treatment for the Menopausal and Post-Menopausal Person.

12. Zung, W.W.K., Rogers, J. and Krugman (1968) Effect of Electroconvulsive Therapy on Memory in Depressive Disorders, in Recent Advances of Biological Psychiatry, Wortis, J., ed., Plenum Press, New York, 160-178, Vol. 10.

13. Obrist, W., Thompson, H., King, C. and Wang, H.S. (1967) Determination of Regional Cerebral Blood Flow by Inhalation of 133-Xenon, Circ. Res., 20, 124-135.

EXPERIMENTAL STUDIES ON CENTROPHENOXINE IN AGING BRAIN

KALIDAS NANDY, M.D., Ph.D.
Geriatric Research, Education and Clinical Center, Veterans Administration
Hospital, Bedford, Massachusetts and Boston University Medical School, Boston,
Massachusetts, USA

INTRODUCTION

Centrophenoxine is a drug unrelated to any other known pharmacological

agents. It was synthesized in French National Scientific Research Center by

Doctors G. Thuillier and P. Rumpf in 1962 and the detailed pharmacology was

studied by Thuillier in the French National Hygiene Institute. The drug was

synthesized by a combination of an amino-alcohol, dimethylamino-ethanol and

p-chlorophenoxyacetic acid. The former component is a natural substance of

animal body and is the immediate precursor of choline which takes part in

membrane biosynthesis by forming phosphatidyl choline, as well as in the

synthesis of the neurotransmitter, acetylcholine. The latter ingredient is,

on the other hand, a synthetic substance chemically related to the plant

hormone, 'auxin', with many of the characteristic properties of the natural

growth factor[1].

A number of clinical studies have been made on this drug on geriatric

patients with the symptoms of confusion and disturbances of concentration

and memory, and significant improvements were reported after several weeks

of treatment [2-11]. Centrophenoxine was found to produce clinical improvements

in 7 out of 30 patients with senile psychosis in a double-blind crossover

study[12]. The detailed clinical studies have been discussed in a separate

chapter in this book. In this chapter, the results of the more experimental

studies on centrophenoxine on aging nerve tissue both in vivo and in vitro

have been discussed.

CENTROPHENOXINE ON LEARNING AND MEMORY

The effects of centrophenoxine on learning and memory of aged mice were studied and the results were correlated with morphological changes in the brain. Twenty old (11-12 months) female mice were treated with the drug at a dose of 100 mg/kg of body weight daily by intraperitoneal injection for three months. The results were compared with control young (3-4 months) and control old mice (11-12 months) injected daily with normal saline. All three groups of animals were deprived of water for the whole day and were only supplied with water ad libitum for two minutes at the end of the daily experiment. Mice were trained in a T-maze and were given 60 seconds to choose the correct side of the maze containing the water bottle. Each animal was given three trials each day and six consecutive correct responses were considered as meeting the criterion. The number of trials required to meet the criterion was recorded for each mouse in all groups. When all mice reached the criterion, the water bottles were shifted to the opposite side of the maze and the number of trials required to attain the criterion were again recorded.

It was observed that the young mice learned with fewer trials than old mice and there was no significant difference between the treated and untreated old mice. However, following the shifting of the water bottle to the opposite side, the treated old mice did significantly better than the aged-matched controls. The young mice did equally well in both cases[13].

CENTROPHENOXINE ON LIFE SPAN

The long-term effect of centrophenoxine on mean and maximum life span of C57BL/6 female mice were studied in our and other laboratories. Fifty animals (6 months old) were treated daily with the drug and another fifty without treatment acted as controls. After 30 months, 20 mice in the treated group and only 5 in the control group survived (x^2 = 10.45, p $>$ 0.002). The study indicated a significant extension of median life span, although the

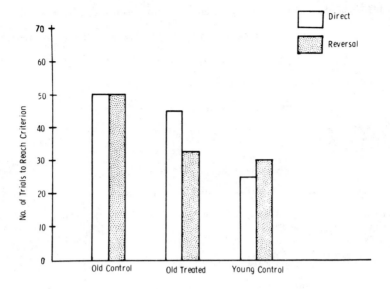

Fig. 1. Average number of trials required to attain criterion in old control, young control, and centrophenoxine-treated old mice.

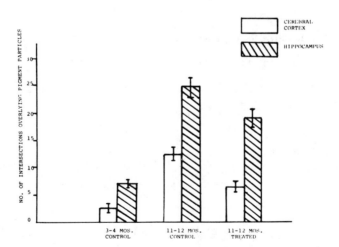

Fig. 2. Histogram showing amounts of lipofuscin pigment in the neurons of the cerebral cortex and hippocampus in control mice aged 3-4 months, control mice aged 11-12 months, and experimental mice aged 11-12 months treated for 3 months with centrophenoxine.

maximum life span was not altered[14]. Hochschild[15] also studied the effect of
the drug on median, mean and maximum survival time of male Swiss Webster
Albino mice and observed an extension by 29.5 percent, 27.3 percent and 39.7
percent respectively. It was suggested that the drug probably exerted its
effects of stabilizing lysosomal and other cellular membranes.

EFFECTS ON LIPOFUSCIN

At the completion of the learning experiments the animals were sacrificed
and lipofuscin pigment in the neurons was quantitated. The pigment was
visualized in frozen sections by its characteristic autofluorescence, histochemical stainings and also be electron microscopy. The pigment was
particularly studied in two regions of the brain, frontal cerebral cortex and
hippocampus in different groups. An age-related increase in the pigment was
noted in the neurons of both regions and significant reduction was observed in
the treated animals after three months of treatment. Ultrastructurally,
lipofuscin appeared to be broken into smaller particules with more numerous
vacuoles within the pigment mass in the treated animals[13]. Neither the
precise significance of the pigment in the neurons nor the mode of action
of the drug are clear in this study.

The effects of the drug on the lipofuscin and metabolic enzymes were
studied in the neurons of CNS of guinea pigs in order to understand the
possible mechanism of action of centrophenoxine. Old guinea pigs (3 years)
were treated with the drug by daily injection for 4 months. A significant
reduction in the lipofuscin pigment in the neurons of cerebral cortex, brain
stem nuclei and spinal cord was observed. This was also associated with a
reduction of succinic dehydrogenase, cytochrome oxidase and lactate dehydrogenase and an increase in the activity of glucose-6-phosphate dehydrogenase
in these neurons by histochemical methods. Different metabolic enzymes were
also studied in degenerating and regenerating neurons in the spinal cord

following axonal injury. The pattern of enzymatic changes seen in those
nerve cells were similar to those in the neurons of the treated guinea pigs.
A diversion of the metabolism of glucose from Krebs cycle to pentose shunt
was observed in the neurons in both cases[16-21]. Since the neurons in the
treated animals exhibited enzymatic changes similar to those in the regenerating neurons of the spinal cord, the reduction of lipofuscin caused by
centrophenoxine was interpreted as an evidence of regeneration in the
treated mice.

The question whether centrophenoxine can prevent lipofuscin formation
if the treatment started very early before the onset of pigmentogensis was
also studied in mice in our laboratory. One month old mice were treated
daily for eleven months, and mice of the same age and sex without treatment
acted as controls. Animals were sacrificed following 2, 5, 8 and 11 months
of treatment and lipofuscin pigment was quantitated using histochemical and
fluorescence methods. Although the pigment formation was consistently
reduced by the treatment for 5 months or more, centrophenoxine did not
prevent pigment formation in these neurons of CNS in the treated animals[22].

The effects of centrophenoxine on the lipofuscin pigments in the CNS
of old rats after treatment for 8 weeks was studied by Riga and Riga[23].
The lipofuscinolytic activity of the drug varied in different regions of
CNS. The reduction were 42.31% in pontine reticular formation, 42.0% in
cerebral cortex layer V cells, 38.9% in overall cerebral cortex, 27.7% in
Purkinje cells. Several studies were also reported by different investigators on the mode of action of the drug on neuronal lipofuscin. Chemnitius
et al[24] studied the effect of the drug on the pigment in the ganglion cells
of the nucleus reticularis gigantocellularis of albino rats using light
microscopy and found a similar change in the pigment. Meier and Glees[25]
studied the effects of the drug on the neurons and satellite cells in the
cervical spinal ganglia by electron microscopy. These authors noted a

TABLE I

LIPOFUSCIN PIGMENT COUNTED BY OCULAR GRID METHOD IN THE NEURONS OF CEREBRAL CORTEX AND HIPPOCAMPUS OF MICE TREATED WITH CENTROPHENOXINE AND AGE-MATCHED CONTROLS

Control group			Treated group		
Age (months)	Neurons of frontal cortex	Neurons of hippocampus	Neurons of frontal cortex	Neurons of hippocampus	Duration of treatment (months)
1	0.4 ± 0.34	0.6 ± 0.66	–	–	–
3	4.80 ± 0.34	6.96 ± 1.08	2.96 ± 0.98* (P = 0.4)	4.76 ± 1.60* (P = 0.2)	2
6	10.12 ± 0.94	14.04 ± 1.08	5.32 ± 0.70* (P = 0.05)	8.68 ± 1.10* (P = 0.05)	5
9	13.02 ± 2.11	19.84 ± 3.68	6.92 ± 0.79* (P = 0.05)	12.24 ± 2.17* (P = 0.05)	8
12	16.04 ± 1.54	23.68 ± 3.40	8.68 ± 1.08	14.04 ± 2.10	11

*The values of P as indicated for the treated group represent the significance level of the statistical difference between the lipofuscin in the neurons of control and treated mice of the same age after variable periods of treatment.
Five mice were sacrificed each time in both treated and control groups.
Ten sections were studied in both frontal cortex and hippocampus of each animal.

disintegration of the pigment masses into smaller particles in the neurons and a final disappearance was seen after increasing periods of treatment. On the other hand, the satellite cells appeared to contain more and more of the pigment and the possibility of removal of the pigment by these cells from the neurons was suggested by these authors. Hasan et al[26,27] made further observations on the possible mode of lipofuscinolytic action of centrophenoxine in the neurons of CNS including hypothalamus of guinea pigs. These authors observed pigment particles in the pericytes and in the endothelial cells of the treated animals. Vacuolated pigment granules were often noted in large spaces within in the capillary endothelium of the animals treated for 35 days and more. The number of vacuoles in the endothelial cells also appeared to increase following prolonged treatment. These authors suggested that the

endothelium probably participates in the removal of the pigment following
breakdown into smaller particles. Further, Spoerri and Glees[28] demonstrated
elimination of the pigment granules to the extracellular space by means of
cytoplasmic protrusions in addition to the removal by the phagocytic cells.

TISSUE CULTURE STUDIES

Tissue culture model has been used in aging studies by number of investigators[28-35]. Several studies have been carried out in our laboratory on the
effect of the drug in vitro using C1300 mouse neuroblastoma cells. These
cells are capable of dividing indefinitely in optimum media and aging
changes are not seen. However, the inhibition of the cell division by the
addition of certain agents such as papaverine, cAMP, prostaglandin E_1, in the
culture media led to the differentiation of these cells. Lipofuscin pigment

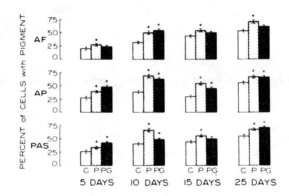

FIG. 3. Effects of 1.1×10^{-5} M papaverine (P) and 5.6×10^{-5} M
prostaglandin E_1 (PG) on pigment formation in T59 neuroblastoma cells
growing on coverslips. Exposure to drugs was started 1 day after
plating. AF means autofluorescence, AP means acid phosphatase, and
PAS means periodic acid schiff stain. The details of the histochemical
procedures are described in the Methods section. The height of each
bar represents the mean of between 40 and 80 counts for 2 to 4
experiments; the bracketed bars represent standard errors, and the
asterisks indicate significant difference from control (C) at the
p   0.05 level.

254

was demonstrated for the first time in these cells in culture following differentiation by histochemical, fluorescence and EM methods. The percent of the cells containing pigment increased with time when the cells were maintained in culture. Additionally, resumption of the cell division by omission of these agents in the media was accompanied by a reduction in the amount of the pigment (Fig. 3)[41].

When centrophenoxine was added to the culture media in the concentration of 1.0 or 3.4 x 10^{-4}M the pigment formation was markedly reduced in these cells without significantly altering the cell viability or cell growth (Table 2)[42]. The results of the studies using histochemical and fluorescence methods were later confirmed by electron microscopy in our laboratory[43]. Spoerri and Glees[44] studied the effects of the drug on the pigment in cultured spinal ganglia neurons and satellite cells. The lipofuscin accumulation occurred in the cytoplasm of the spinal ganglia neurons in vitro similar to those in vivo during 1-4 weeks in culture. The pigment was seen as osmio-philic bodies of different sizes and shapes within the mitochondria enclosed in a double unit membrane. On addition of centrophenoxine in the culture media the vacuolation and breakdown of the pigment were seen similar to those in animals. Osmiophilic granules were seen also in the satellite cells investing the neurons. The pigment granules with vacuoles were demonstrated in the periphery of the neurons and satellite cells prior to their removal from the nerve cells. Cytoplasmic processes of the neurons filled with pigment were also frequently seen. It was suggested that both the cytoplasmic processes and the satellite cells were responsible for the presence of pigment in the extracellular space. An active uptake of the pigment granules were seen in the proliferating endothelial cells of the residual capillaries[28]. The removal of the pigment was also associated with hypertrophy and the prominence of the rough endoplasmic reticulum in the nerve cells. Although the significance of this change is not clear, an evidence of increased protein synthesis was suggested.

Table 1. Effect of Centrophenoxine on the Percentage of T59 Neuroblastoma Cells, Growing on Glass Coverslips, Which Contain Pigment [a].

Treatment	Fluorescence	APase	PAS
Regular media	33 ± 2*	59 ± 2*	70 ± 3*
Papaverine	51 ± 4	87 ± 1	88 ± 1
Papaverine + centrophenoxine (10^{-4}M)	45 ± 3	28 ± 2*	27 ± 3*
Papaverine + centrophenoxine (3.4×10^{-4}M)	28 ± 3*	29 ± 2*	34 ± 3*

[a] Papaverine was present at 1.1×10^{-5}M for 9 days starting on day 9 after plating; in the centrophenoxine-treated cultures centrophenoxine was also added on day 9 and continued for an additional 9 days. Media were changed everyday. The numbers are means ± standard errors, and an asterisk indicates a value which is different from papaverine treatment at $p < .001$ level. See methods section for details of procedures.

SIGNIFICANCE OF LIPOFUSCIN PIGMENT AND CENTROPHENOXINE TREATMENT

Despite numerous reports on the lipofuscin pigment in the literature on its various aspects, information on two most fundamental questions, namely its mode of origin and physiopathologic significance, are surprisingly lacking[44-68]. The investigators seem to differ widely in their views on the genesis of the pigment. The pigment appear to be derived from one or more of the organelles within the cell. The generally accepted notion has been in favor of the lysosomal origin of the pigment. The strong acid phosphatase activity and the striking ultrastructural similarity between the two are the major evidences for this hypothesis[13, 18, 45]. Biochemical isolation of the pigment from the brain samples followed by electron microscopy provide further evidence in support of this hypothesis[66, 67].

The arguments have also been made in favor of the possible origin of the pigment from the mitochondria by Hess[69] and Roizin[70]. Hasan and Glees[71] observed that the pigment formation might be preceded by an increased concentration and clumping of mitochondria resulting in the disturbance of normal metabolic activity. This latter condition might lead to the accumulation of insoluble fatty acids which are introduced in the pigment formation[72, 73]. These authors have further extended the work to the lipofuscin formation in tissue culture with similar observations.

It is difficult at this time to make any definite statement on the origin of this pigment. The available evidences in the literature tend to indicate that the origin of the pigment may take place from a variety of intracellular organelles and cell membranes which have undergone wear and tear and deterioration during aging. The final breakdown of the materials probably takes place in the lysosomes where these are segregated in an attempt to metabolize and probably reutilize the materials[74].

There are numerous reports in the literature to indicate that lipofuscin is found in the nondividing cells, which are more likely to show the effects of aging[18, 45, 46, 47, 71]. Recent studies in our laboratory using mouse neuroblastoma cells in culture have provided further evidences along this line. These tumor cells are capable of dividing indefinitely under optimum conditions in tissue culture, but exhibit properties of normal neurons if division is arrested by chemicals such as papaverine, cyclic AMP or prostaglandin E_1. However, when these agents were omitted in the culture media, the cells resumed their dividion. It was observed that the differentiated neuroblastoma cells show aging changes like normal neurons in the animals and develop lipofuscin pigment. On the other hand, omission of the differentiating agents in the media was associated with the resumption of cell division and marked reduction in the pigment formation[41]. Those experiments provided further confirmation on the positive correlation between cell differentiation

and lipofuscin formation. Several intriguing questions may still be raised.
Why do non-dividing cells accumulate the pigment unlike the mitotic cells?
Why does lipofuscin pigment accumulate in the neurons of older animals
but not in the young? What happen to the cells treated with the drug? It
may, however, be speculated that the cells in the young animals may have the
special ability to metabolize or reutilize the products of intracellular wear
and tear, whicy might be lost during aging. For example, a change or loss
certain lysosomal enzymes might take place during the life time of animals and
this might account for the accumulation in the old neurons of partially
digested or undigested cellular residue or "garbage" as lipofuscin pigment.

The understanding on the functional significance of the pigment in the
neurons is even more lacking. While some investigators think that the pigment
might be harmful to the cells, others are in favor of its beneficial effects.
This confusion may partly be due to the lack of direct evidences on the
functions of the cells with and without the pigment. Ideally, studies should
be carried out on the functional properties of the cells before and after
the formation of pigment as well as following the removal of the pigment by
drugs. The studies by Nandy[13], and Nandy and Lal[21], showed a significant
improvement of learning and memory in mice following centrophenoxine treatment,
which was also associated with a reduction in lipofuscin in the neurons of
cerebral cortex and hippocampus. On the other hand, Lal et al[55] demonstrated
that rats subjected to vitamin E deficient diet showed a deterioration of
the learning and memory and an increase in the lipofuscin pigment in the
neurons of the cerebral cortex and hippocampus. It may, therefore, be
argued that a relation between lipofuscin formation and neuronal function
might exist. Although there is no direct evidence to indicate that lipofuscin is harmful or toxic to the cells, it appears reasonable to assume that
the process of wear and tear, underlying pigmentogenesis might be detrimental
to the cullular functions. Lipofuscin may, therefore, represent the

product of the damage rather than a causative factor. On the other hand, the accumulation of large amounts of the pigment occupying a substantial part of the cell soma might also be detrimental to smooth functional operations within the cells.

It is not clear from the various studies how exactly the treatment with centrophenoxine exerts its beneficial effects. The reduction of the pigment might be one of several ways the drug might act. Although the earlier studies indicated that the drug removes already formed pigment, more recent studies tend to offer evidence more in favor of a reduction of the rate of pigment formation. It appears reasonable to assume that both removal of cellular garbage as well as reduction of intracellular wear and tear as caused by the drug might be beneficial to cellular functions. There are also evidences that the drug stimulates ribosomal RNA synthesis and also diverts the metabolism of glucose from via Krebs cycle to pentose shunt. Since these changes have been frequently observed in areas tissue regeneration, it may be suggested that centrophenoxine exerts its action by setting up some regenerative changes in the cells probably by stimulation of the metabolic processes.

Summary:

Centrophenoxine is a new drug which has been found clinically beneficial to patients with the symptoms of senile dementia in Europe. Animal studies following daily treatment of mice produced improvements of learning and memory as well as a reduction of lipofuscin pigment in the neurons of frontal cortex and hippocampus. The longterm treatment with the drug also provided some evidence in favor of extension of the mean lifespan of mice. The effects of the drug also have been reproduced in other rodents including guinea pigs and rats. Tissue culture studies revealed that the drug is capable of reducing lipofuscin formation both in mouse neuroblastoma cells in culture as well as in brain explants. The significance of lipofuscin pigment has been discussed and it has been suggested that drug probably acts by stimulating cellular

metabolism and regenerative changes.

REFERENCES:

1. Thuillier, G., Rumpff, R., and Thuillier, J. (1959) Compt. Rend. Soc. Biol. Paris, 153, 1914.
2. Destrem, H. (1961) Presse Med., 69, 1999.
3. Delay, J., Thuillier, J., Pichot, P. (1960) Ann. Medicopsychol., 118, 133.
4. Fichez, L. F., Boureq, G. and Nedelec, G. (1961) Gaz. Hop. Paris, 133, 1137.
5. Coirault, R. (1959) Rev. Lyon. Med., 179.
6. Coirault, R. Desclos de la Fonchais, S. (1959) Gaz. Hop., 131, 1151.
7. Coirault, R. (1960) Soc. de Pathol. Comparee, Rev. pathol. gen et physiol. clin., 60, 451.
8. Coirault, R. (1960) Ann. med.-psych., 118(1), 119.
9. Coirault, R. Rouif, G., Pourpre, H., Damasio, R., Deligne, P., David, M., Talairach, J. (1960) Presse med., 68, 215.
10. Coirault, R., Deligne, P., Rouif, J. (1960) Agressologie, 1, 113.
11. Coirault, R. (1960) Gaz. Hop., 132, 701.
12. Denber, H.C.B., Meshal, E., Tellez, D.N. and Richman (1964) Dis. Nerv. Syst., 25, 724.
13. Nandy, K. (1978) Am. Ger. Soc., XXVI, 74.
14. Nandy, K. and Lal, H. (1978) in Neuro-psychopharmacology, Deniker, P., Villeneuve, C.R.A. ed., Pergamon Press, New York, pp. 1633-1645.
15. Hochschile, R. (1973) J. Exp. Gerontol. 8, 177.
16. Nandy, K. and Bourne, G.H. (1966) Nature, 210, 313.
17. Nandy, K. (1968) J. Gerontol. 23, 82.
18. Nandy, K. (1971) Acta Neuropath., 19, 25.
19. Nandy, K. and Bourne, G.H. (1964) Archiev. Neurol., 11, 547.
20. Nandy, K. (1969) in Motor Neuron Disease, Norris, F. ed. Grune and Stratton, Inc., pp. 319-334.
21. Nandy, K. (1978) in Senile Dementia: A Biomedical Approach, Nandy, K. ed., Elsevier North-Holland, New York, pp. 19-32.
22. Nandy, K. (1978) Mech. Age. Dev., 8, 131.
23. Riga, S. and Riga, D. (1974) Brain Res., 72, 265.
24. Chemnitius K-HV, Machnik, G., Low, O. (1970) Exp. Path. 4, 163.
25. Meier, C. and Glees, P. (1971) Acta Neuropath., 17, 310.
26. Hasan, M., Glees, P. and Spoerri, P.E. (1974) Cell Tissue Res., 150, 369.
27. Hasan, M., Glees, P. and El-Ghazzawi, E. (1974) Exp. Gerontol., 9, 153.
28. Spoerri, P.E. and Glees, P. (1973) Exp. Gerontol., 8, 259.
29. Smith, J.R. and Hayflick, I. (1974) J. Cell Biol., 62, 48.
30. Cristofalo, V.J. and Kritchevsky, D. (1969) Med. Exp., 19, 313.
31. Cristofalo, V.J. and Kritchevsky, D. (1966) J. Cell.Comp. Physiol., 67, 125.
32. Cristofalo, V.J. (1972) Adv. Gerontol. Res., 4, 45.
33. Cristofalo, V.J., Kabakjian, J.R., Kritchevsky, D. (1967) Proc. Soc. Exp. Biol. Med., 126, 648.
34. Bell, E., Marek, L.F., Levinstone, D.S., Merrill, C., Sher, S., Young, I.T. and Eden, M. (1978) Science, 202, 1158.
35. Deamer, D.W., and Gonzales, J. (1964) Arch. Biochem. Biophys., 165, 421.
36. Prasad, K.N., Gilmer, K., and Kumar, S. (1973) Proc. Soc. Exp. Med. Biol., 143, 1168.
37. Glazer, R.I., and Schneider, F.H. (1975) J. Biol. Chem., 250, 2745.

38. Phillips, H.J. (1973) in Tissue Culture: Methods and Applications, Academic Press, New York, pp. 402-406
39. Lowry, O., Rosebrough, N., Farr, A., and Randall, J. (1951) J. Biol. Chem., 193, 265.
40. Seeds, N.W., Gilman, A.G., Amano, T., and Nirenberg, M.W. (1970) Proc. Natl. Acad. Sci., 66, 160.
41. Nandy, K. and Schneider, F.H. (1976) in Neurobiology of Aging, Terry, R. and Gershon, S. ed., Raven Press, New York, pp. 245-264.
42. Schneider, F.H. and Nandy, K. (1977) J. Geront., 32, 132.
43. Nandy, K., Baste, C. and Schneider, F.H. (1978) Exp. Geront., 13, 311.
44. Spoerri, P.E. and Glees, P. (1974) Mech. Age. Dev., 3, 131.
45. Samorajski, T., Keefe, J.R. and Ordy, J.M. (1964) J. Gerontol., 19, 262.
46. Samorajski, T., Ordy, J.M. and Keefe, J.R. (1965) J. Cell Biol., 26, 779.
47. Brody, H. (1960) J. Gerontol., 16, 258.
48. Hasan, M. and Glees, P. (1972) Gerontologia, 18, 217.
49. Nanda, B.A. and Getty, R. (1974) Current Res., I, 11.
50. Whiteford, R. and Getty R. (1966) J. Gerontol., 21, 31.
51. Brizzee, K.R., Ordy, J.M, Hansche, J. (1976) in Neurobiology of Aging, R. Terry and Gershon, S. ed., Raven Press, New York, pp. 229-244.
52. Sekhon, S.S. and Maxwell, D.S. (1974) J. Neurocytol., 3, 59.
53. Weglicki, W.B., Reichel, W. and Nair, P.P. (1966) J. Gerontol., 21, 469.
54. Sulkin, N.M. and Srivanji, P. (1960) J. Gerontol., 15, 2.
55. Lal, H., Pogacar, S., Daly, P.R. and Puri, S.K. (1973) in Neurobiological Aspects of Maturation and Aging, Ford, D. ed., New York, Elsevier North-Holland, pp. 129=140.
56. Hamprel, H. (1934) Arch. Path. Anat. Physiol. 327, 112.
57. Bomer, S. (1929) Acta Dermat. Veterol., 10, 391.
58. Jayne, E.P. (1950) J. Gerontol., 5, 318.
59. Hendley, D.D., Mildvan, A.S., Reporter, M.C. (1963) J. Gerontol., 18, 144.
60. Hendley, D.D., Mildvan, A.S., Reporter, M.C. (1963) 18, 250.
61. Brody, H. (1955) J. Comp. Neurol., 102, 511.
62. Sulkin, N.M. (1955) J. Comp. Neurol., 102, 511.
63. Sulkin, N.M. (1958) Anat. Rec., 130, 377.
64. Gedigk, P. and Bontke, E. (1956) Z. Zellforsch., 44, 495.
65. O'Steen, K.W. and Nandy, K. (1970) Am. J. Anat., 128, 359.
66. Siakotos, A.N., Watanaba, I., Siato, A. Biochem. Med., 4, 361.
67. Siakotos, A.N., Goebel, H.H., Patel, V. (1972) Adv. Exp. Med. & Biol., 19, 53.
68. Reichel, W. and Garcia-Bunuel, R. (1970) Am. J. Clin. Path., 53, 243.
69. Hess, A. (1955) Anat. Rec., 123, 399.
70. Roizin, L. (1964) J. Neuropathol. Exp. Neurol., 23, 209.
71. Hasan, M. and Glees, P. (1972) Gerontologia, 18, 217.
72. Gopinath, G. and Glees, P. (1974) Acta. Anat., 89, 14.
73. Glees, P. and Gopinath, G. Z. Zellforsch, 141, 285.
74. Brody, H. and Vijayashanker, N. (1978) in Handbook of the Biology of Aging, Finch, C.E. and Hayflick, L., ed. Van Nostrand, New York, Vol. 1, pp. 343-384.

EFFECTS OF CENTROPHENOXIN ON CEREBRAL CIRCULATION
IN GERIATRIC PATIENTS

SIEGFRIED HOYER, M.D.
Department of Pathochemistry and General Neurochemistry,
University of Heidelberg, D-6900 Heidelberg,FRG

Centrophenoxin can be assigned to the group of stimulant drugs
because of its chemical structure. It is known as a nootropic
agent in gerontopsychiatry. In vivo investigations in experimental
animals showed a marked increase of the glucose transfer from the
arterial blood across the blood-brain barrier into the brain
tissue under centrophenoxin. However, this increase was not due to
a general increase of the permeability of the blood-brain barrier
(65,66). In vitro experiments in brain slices demonstrated an increase of the aerobic glycolysis and the respiration of the
nervous tissue under centrophenoxin which was attributed to an
activation of cerebral glucose metabolism which was about 20% as
compared to control conditions (36). First investigations on the
effect of centrophenoxin on disturbed brain functions in patients
suffering from organic brain syndromes were reported in the
1960's (90). Centrophenoxin was said to be effective in patients
suffering from agitation, lack of social contacts, lack of drive,
depression and cognitive defect due to organic brain diseases of
various etiologies (19,75,95). Further clinical investigations
in 200 patients mostly suffering from presenile or senile encephalopathies and less from brain infarctions or cerebral hemorrhages
showed positive results under a two-to-three week treatment with
centrophenoxin. About 70% of the patients suffering from presenile
or senile encephalopathies improved under centrophenoxin; in about
30% of the cases this therapy was not successful although the
patients did not deteriorate. In patients with brain infarctions
and cerebral hemorrhages the rate of improvement was about 60%
under centrophenoxin treatment (77). Though the clinical studies
mentioned did not fulfil strict criteria for a clinico-pharmaco-
logical investigation (no double-blind study, no control groups,
no precise clinical diagnosis etc) these clinical data and the

experimental results mentioned indicate that centrophenoxin may have a positive effect on the disturbances in cerebral blood flow and/or oxidative metabolism of the brain which are associated with cerebral diseases such as stroke or dementia. Results of investigations in these diseases will be dealt with here in more detail. However, some important points concerning brain blood flow and metabolism under physiological and pathophysiological conditions, i.e. in organic brain disorders, will be discussed first.

Physiological aspects

The normal adult brain weighs about 1400 g on average, i.e. 2-3% of the total normal body weight. In spite of its relatively small weight, the energy-needs of this organ are extremely high. In 24 hours the normal adult brain is perfused by about 1000 l of blood which is about 20% of the cardiac output. In the same time the brain consumes about 70 l of oxygen which is also about 20% of the oxygen consumption of the whole body. In a 24-hour period the brain takes up about 100 g of glucose which is about 25% of the normal carbohydrate uptake per day. These data may illustrate the predominant role of the brain in the body as a whole.

Two main factors ensure that the enormously high supply of the brain with blood and substrates is maintained. These are the cerebral perfusion pressure and the partial pressure of CO_2 in the arterial blood ($paCO_2$). The cerebral perfusion pressure is calculated as the difference of mean arterial blood pressure and intracranial pressure. In the case of a normal intracranial pressure only the relationship between mean arterial blood pressure and cerebral blood flow is of importance.

This pressure/flow relationship is well known as autoregulation of cerebral blood flow which remains undisturbed within the ranges of mean arterial blood pressure of 50 to 150 mm Hg (10,11,16,17, 30,32,33,46,52,57,58,59,62,72,84,85,86,94).Within these limits both, the oxidative and energy metabolism of the brain seem to remain unchanged (46,53,82,83,96).

Cerebral blood flow changes with $paCO_2$. In arterial hypocapnia cerebral blood flow falls, whereas it increases in arterial hypercapnia (CO_2 reactivity of the cerebral vessels)(2,3,4,6,21,31,34, 39,55,56,58,61,71,72,74,78,79,80,91,92).However, the cerebral metabolic rates of oxygen and glucose remain constant in the ranges of $paCO_2$ of 15 to about 80 mm Hg. And so does cerebral energy metabolism (2,3,5,12,13,18,24,25,26,27,28,81).

Under normal conditions the brain uses only glucose to obtain energy (20,23,40). Glucose enters the brain by means of a facilitated transport mechanism across the blood-brain barrier. Only about 5% of the total amount of glucose used in the brain diffuses across the blood-brain barrier under normal conditions (8,9,15,63, 67,68,70). In the brain cells glucose is metabolized via the Embden-Meyerhof pathway and the tricarboxylic acid cycle which is extended by a γ-aminobutyric acid (GABA) shunt and an amino acid pool (76).

There is no doubt that normally a close relationship exists between cerebral blood flow on the one hand and both, oxidative and energy metabolism of the brain on the other. Under pathological conditions such as dementia or stroke this relationship can be interfered with and glucose transport across the blood-brain barrier and/or glucose breakdown in the brain cell can be disturbed (50).

Pathophysiological aspects

The most important brain diseases in middle-aged and elderly patients are dementia and stroke. Stroke may be primarily due to rheological factors while dementia may be primarily due to a disease in the brain tissue itself.

In detail, the main factors producing rheological disturbances may be abnormalities in arterial blood pressure, mostly arterial hypertension, arteriosclerosis or thrombosis of the larger cerebral vessels, cerebral embolism, cardiac failure and increasing blood viscosity. These basically extracerebral diseases produce disturbances (mostly decreases) in regional cerebral blood flow which lead to focal brain damage, i.e. clinically to a primary neurological deficit and secondarily to a dementia. Therefore a treatment should primarily be directed towards eliminating the extracerebral causes of cerebral infarctions. Additional to this therapy it would seem to be necessary to treat the perifocal brain edema and the regionally disturbed brain blood flow (and metabolism), too. However, the treatment of the disturbed cerebral blood flow by

means of the so-called vasoactive drugs is very problematical
since most of these drugs do not influence cerebral blood flow at
all (22,37,44,69; further literature in each of these references).

In dementia about 90% of the patients show morphologically
either degenerative (Alzheimer) variations, or cerebrovascular
(multi infarct) variations (in smaller vessels of the brain) or
both kinds of variations. In 60% of them dementia was due to degenerative changes, in 20 to 25% due to cerebrovascular variations
and in 15 to 20% due to both disturbances (51,89). From a nosological point of view, "simple" senile dementia, Alzheimer's senile
and Alzheimer's presenile dementias are variations of the same
degenerative brain disease (1,7,14,54,60,64,87,88). Based on a
psychometric ischemic score it is possible to differentiate between the degenerative and the cerebrovascular type of dementia
(29,35,45). The two large different dementia types reflect in different patterns of brain blood flow and oxydative metabolism. In
the degenerative group both, cerebral blood flow and CMR-oxygen
were in a nearly normal range on average while in the multi infarct
group both parameters were decreased on average. A similar clearcut
correlation could not be found for CMR-glucose (49). As far as
cerebral blood flow was concerned Hachinski et al. came to same
results (29). Another factor which influences brain blood flow
and metabolism in dementia patients is the duration of the dementia
process. In the initial phase of the disease (duration of the disease less than two years) both cerebral blood flow and CMR-oxygen
were not markedly disturbed in either degenerative or multi infarct
dementia, whereas CMR-glucose was decreased in the degenerative
and increased in the vascular group. In the intermediate phase of
the dementia process (duration of the disease between two and ten
years) cerebral blood flow, CMR-oxygen and CMR-glucose decreased
in both types of dementia. In chronic dementia (duration of the
disease longer than ten years) brain blood flow and metabolism
stabilized at a common pathologically low level in both dementia
types. Cerebral blood flow and metabolism seem to be as high as
the needs of the brain (42,43).

Further points in dementia which must be considered when esti-
mating the variations in brain blood flow and metabolism are the

degree and the kind of psychiatric impairment. In patients suffering from mild to moderate dementia, the parameters brain blood
flow and metabolism were only mildly or moderately decreased. In
severely demented patients no correlations could be found between
the degree of psychiatric impairment in dementia and the degree
of decreases in cerebral blood flow and metabolism. There was,
however, a clear correlation between the deranged functional state
of the brain and its disturbed blood flow and metabolism (48).

It would thus seem that basically at least three factors -
the type of dementia, the duration of dementia and the kind of
psychiatric impairment - might influence the quality and the quantity of the variations in brain blood flow and metabolism. There
is no doubt that these different factors might interfere with
each other and might thus produce a larger number of factors determining the disturbances of brain blood flow and metabolism in
dementia.

Two more points should, however, be considered generally in the
drug treatment of dementia symptoms and its estimation:
1.)The above mentioned differences in the quality and the quantity
of the variations of brain blood flow and metabolism may be of
etiological significance at least as far as the different disturbances in the morphological variations are concerned. It is therefore more than doubtful whether a single drug would be able to
counteract all disturbances of brain blood flow and metabolism
in all cases of dementia. Results on improvements of cerebral
blood flow and/or metabolism and the clinical symptoms showing a
success rate of 50 to 60% after a treatment of several days or
weeks are much more convincing and could also be explained in
pathophysiological terms. Drugs which act on brain blood flow
and/or metabolism and clinical symptoms and of which almost 100%
positive effects on these parameters are claimed should be treated
with much skepticism.
2.)A spontaneous improvement of cerebral blood flow and metabolism
accompanied by an improvement of the dementia symptoms could be
observed in about one third of the patients within three weeks
while in the remaining two thirds both biological and clinical
parameters deteriorated more and more (41). It would thus seem
to be of general importance in the treatment of dementia symptoms

and of disturbed brain blood flow and metabolism with "vasoactive"
or "metabolic-active" drugs that the information contained in the
above results be taken into account in the interests of successful
therapy.

Effects of centrophenoxin on regional and global cerebral blood flow and on oxidative brain metabolism in patients with stroke and dementia

There are two clinical-experimental studies in which the effects
of centrophenoxin on regional cerebral blood flow and on global
brain blood flow and metabolism were investigated.

Herrschaft et al. measured regional cerebral blood flow by
means of the intra-arterial ^{133}Xenon-clearance method in 18 patients suffering from mild to moderate neurological deficits such
as hemiparesis, aphasia, apraxia etc. mostly due to an arteriosclerosis of the larger cerebral vessels. They found an 11.4%
increase of the cerebral grey matter flow 15 min after an intravenous application of 1000 mg centrophenoxin. This increase was
statistically significant as compared to resting values. The cerebral white matter flow was not influenced by centrophenoxin. The
intravenous application of 500 mg centrophenoxin did not show any
effect on cerebral grey matter flow. Herrschaft et al. suggested
that centrophenoxin does not have any effect on cerebral vascu-
lature but might act on oxidative brain metabolism. The increase
in cerebral grey matter flow after application of centrophenoxin
was interpreted as a secondary effect while the primary effect
of centrophenoxin was activation of brain metabolism (38).

Using the modified Kety-Schmidt technique Hoyer and coworkers
(47) studied the influence of centrophenoxin along with piracetam
and extract.sanguin.deprot.sicc. after a three-week treatment
on global cerebral blood flow, CMR-oxygen and CMR-glucose in a
total of 90 patients suffering either from multi infarct dementia,
primary degenerative (Alzheimer) dementia and dementia due to
chronic alcoholism. In a randomized study each drug group comprised 20 patients, 30 patients serving as controls were treated
with an intravenously applied infusion of 500 ml levulose 5% per
day, also over a period of three weeks. It could be shown that
centrophenoxin improved significantly the decreased cerebral

TABLE 1

	age years	resting rate CBF ml/100 g min	CMR-oxygen ml/100 g min	CMR-glucose mg/100g min	after treatment CBF ml/100 min	CMR-oxygen ml/100g min	CMR-glucose mg/100g min
Extr.sanguin. deprot.sicc.							
M.I.; n = 6	71	29.9	2.50	2.69	36.1	2.73	3.50
P.D.; n = 4	63	52.0	3.90	4.83	47.0	3.14	4.93
A.D.; n = 10	47	28.0	1.99	3.03	45.1[+]	3.23[+]	4.14
Centrophenoxin							
M.I.; n = 9	68	33.3	2.50	3.39	47.5[+]	2.92	4.43
P.D.; n = 4	65	32.1	2.36	3.14	37.8	2.25	3.60
A.D.; n = 7	43	50.1	3.62	3.70	37.7	2.40	3.64
Piracetam							
M.I.; n = 7	59	33.3	2.41	3.26	49.5[+]	3.83[+]	4.88[+]
P.D.; n = 4	62	32.3	2.23	3.57	38.3	3.15	3.83
A.D.; n = 9	44	42.1	3.56	4.77	46.2	3.44	4.83

Mean values of cerebral blood flow (CBF), CMR-oxygen and CMR-glucose in patients with organic brain disorders (M.I. = multi infarct dementia; P.D. = primary degenerative dementia; A.D. = dementia due to alcoholism) before and after a three-week treatment with extr.sanguin.deprot.sicc., Centrophenoxin and Piracetam.
+ α = O.O5

blood flow in patients suffering from multi infarct dementia. This
result was in agreement with the findings of Herrschaft et al.
(see above). Centrophenoxin also improved the decreased CMR-glucose in the same group of patients, but this increase of CMR-glucose was just below the level of statistical significance (Table 1).
Effects of centrophenoxin in improving the biological parameters
of the brain in patients suffering from dementia due to Alzheimer's
disease or chronic alcoholism could not be observed. However, it
is necessary to investigate the effect of centrophenoxin on the
variations in the Alzheimer group in a further study since this
group of patients was too small. It should be noted that the significant increase in cerebral blood flow under centrophenoxin in the
multi infarct group was paralled by an improvement of the clinical-
psychiatric parameters. When there was no change or deterioration
of the biological brain parameters, there were generally no
changes or deteriorations in the clinical findings.

To sum up, centrophenoxin may have a positive effect on disturbed cerebral blood flow but its indications seem to be stroke
and multi infarct dementia.

REFERENCES

1. Albert, E. (1964) Senile Demenz und Alzheimer'sche Krankheit
   als Ausdruck des gleichen Krankheitsgeschehens. Fortschr.
   Neurol.Psychiat.32, 625 - 673.
2. Alberti, E., Hoyer, S., Hamer, J., Stoeckel, H., Packschiess,P.,
   Weinhardt, F. (1975) The effect of carbon dioxide on cerebral
   blood flow and cerebral metabolism in dogs. Br.J.Anaesth.47,
   941-947.
3. Alexander, S.C., Cohen, P.J., Wollman, H., Smith, T.C.,
   Reivich, M., van der Molen, R.A.(1965) Cerebral carbohydrate
   metabolism during hypocarbia in man. Studies during nitrous
   oxide anesthesia. Anesthesiology 26, 624 - 632.
4. Alexander, S.C., Marshall, B.E., Agnoli, A.: Cerebral blood
   flow in the goat with sustained hypocapnia. Scand.J.clin.
   Lab.Invest.(Suppl.102) VIII, C.
5. Alexander, S.C., Smith, T.C., Strobel, G., Stephen, G.W.,
   Wollman, H. (1968) Cerebral carbohydrate metabolism of man
   during respiratory and metabolic alkalosis J.appl.Physiol.24,
   66 - 72.
6. Alexander, S.C., Wollman, H., Cohen, P.E., Behar, M.(1964)
   Cerebrovascular response to pa CO_2 during halothane anesthesia
   in man. J. appl.Physiol.19, 561 - 565
7. Arab, A. (1960) Unité nosologique entre démence sénile et
   maladie d'Alzheimer d'après une étude statistique et anatomo-
   clinique. Sist.Nerv.12, 189 - 201.
8. Atkinson, A.J., Weiss, M.F. (1969) Kinetics of blood-cerebro-
   spinal fluid glucose transfer in normal dogs. Amer.J.Physiol.216,
   1120 - 1126.

9. Bachelard, H.S. (1975) How does glucose enter brain cells? In: D.H.Ingvar, N.A.Lassen (Eds.): Brain work. The coupling of function, metabolism and blood flow in the brain. Copenhagen; Munksgaard, pp 126 - 141.

10.Bernsmeier, A.: Durchblutung des Gehirns. In: M.Monnier (Ed.) (1963)Physiologie und Pathophysiologie des vegetativen Nervensystems. Bd.II. Stuttgart; Hippokrates, pp 607 - 640.

11.Carlyle, A., Grayson, J. (1955) Blood pressure and the regulation of brain blood flow. J. Physiol. (Lond.) 127, 15 - 16 P.

12.Cohen, P.J., Alexander, S.C., Wollman, H.: Effects of hypocarbia and of hypoxia with normocarbia on cerebral blood flow and metabolism in man. Scand.J.clin.Lab.Invest.Suppl.102,IV,A.

13.Cohen,P.J., Wollman, H., Alexander, S.C.,Chase, P.E.,Behar,M.G. (1964) Cerebral carbohydrate metabolism in man during halothane anesthesia. Effects of pa CO_2 on some aspects of carbohydrate utilization. Anesthesiology 25, 185 - 191.

14.Constantinidis, J.: Is Alzheimer's disease a major form of senile dementia? Clinical, anatomical and genetic data, in: R.Katzman, R.D.Terry, Katherine L.Bick (Eds.): Alzheimer's disease: Senile dementia and related disorders (Aging Vol.7), New York, Raven Press 1978, pp 15 - 25

15.Crone, C., Thompson, A.M. (1970) Permeability of brain capillaries, in: C.Crone, N.A.Lassen (Eds.): Capillary permeability. Copenhagen; Munksgaard pp 446 - 455

16.Dinsdale, H.B., Robertson, D.M., Haas, R.A. (1974) Cerebral blood flow in acute hypertension. Arch. Neurol. 31, 80 - 87.

17.Ekström-Jodal, B., Häggendal, E., Linder, L.-E., Nilsson,N.J. (1972) Cerebral blood flow autoregulation at high arterial pressures and different levels of carbon dioxide tension in dogs. In: C.Fieschi (Ed.) Cerebral blood flow and intracranial pressure. Basel, München, Paris, London, New York, Sydney; S.Karger, pp 6 - 10

18.Folbergrova, J., MacMillan, V., Siesjö, B.K.(1972) The effect of moderate and marked hypercapnia upon the energy state and upon the cytoplasmatic $NADH/NAD^+$ - ratio of the rat brain. J. Neurochem.19, 2497 - 2505

19.Gerstenbrand,F., Hoff, H., Prosenz, P. (1963) Therapeutische Erfahrungen mit Lucidril bei neuro-psychiatrischen Krankheitsbildern. Wien.med.Wschr. 113, 539 - 543

20.Gibbs, E.L.,Lennox, W.G., Nims, L.F., Gibbs, F.A. (1942) Arterial-venous differences in man. J. biol. Chem. 144, 325 - 332

21.Gotoh, F., Meyer, J.S., Tagaki, Y. (1965) Cerebral effects of hyperventilation in man. Arch. Neurol. 12, 410 - 423

22.Gottstein, U. (1962) Der Hirnkreislauf unter dem Einfluß vasoaktiver Substanzen. Heidelberg; Hüthig

23.Gottstein, U., Bernsmeier, A., Sedlmeyer, J. (1963) Der Kohlenhydratstoffwechsel des menschlichen Gehirns. I. Untersuchungen mit substratspezifischen enzymatischen Methoden bei normaler Hirndurchblutung. Klin.Wschr.41, 943 - 948

24.Gottstein, U., Gabriel, F.H., Held, K., Textor, Th.(1977) Continuous monitoring of arterial and cerebralvenous glucose concentrations in man. Advantage, procedure and results in: Blood glucose monitoring. Methodology and clinical application of continuous in vivo glucose analysis. Stuttgart, Thieme, pp 127 - 135

25. Gottstein, U., Zahn, U., Held, K., Gabriel, F.H., Textor, Th., Berghoff, W. (1976) Einfluß der Hyperventilation auf Hirndurch- blutung und cerebralen Stoffwechsel des Menschen. Untersuchun- gen bei fortlaufender Registrierung der arterio-hirnvenösen Glucosedifferenz. Klin.Wschr. 54, 373 - 381

26. Granholm, L., Lukjanova, L., Siesjö, B.K. (1969) The effect of marked hyperventilation upon tissue levels of NADH, lactate, pyruvate, phosphocreatine and adenosine phosphates of rat brain. Acta physiol. scand.77, 179 - 199

27. Granholm, L., Siesjö, B.K. (1969) The effects of hypercapnia and hypocapnia upon the cerebrospinal fluid lactate and pyru- vate concentrations and upon the lactate, pyruvate, ATP, ADP, phosphocreatine and creatine concentrations of cat brain tissue. Acta physiol.scand. 75, 257 - 266

28. Granholm, L., Siesjö, B.K. (1971) The effect of combined res- piratory and non-respiratory alkalosis on energy metabolites and acid-base parameters in the rat brain. Acta physiol.scand. 81, 307 - 314

29. Hachinski, V.C., Iliff, L.D., Zilkha, E., Du Boulay, G.H., Mc Allister, V.L., Marshall, J., Ross-Russell, R.W., Symon, L. (1975) Cerebral blood flow in dementia. Arch. Neurol. 32, 632 - 637

30. Häggendal, E. (1965) Blood flow autoregulation of the cerebral grey matter with comments on its mechanism. Acta neurol. scand. Suppl. 14, 104 - 110

31. Häggendal, E., Johansson, B. (1965) Effects of arterial carbon dioxide tension and oxygen saturation on cerebral blood flow autoregulation in dogs. Acta physiol. scand. (Suppl. 258) 66, 27 - 53

32. Harper, A.M. (1965) The inter-relationship between ap CO_2 and blood pressure in the regulation of blood flow through the cere- bral cortex. Acta neurol. scand. Suppl. 14, 94 - 103

33. Harper, A.M. (1966) Autoregulation of cerebral blood flow: influence of the arterial blood pressure on the blood flow through the cerebral cortex. J.Neurol. Neurosurg. Psychiat.29, 398 - 403

34. Harper, A.M., Glass, H.J.(1965) Effect of alteration in the arterial carbon dioxide tension on the blood flow through the cerebral cortex at normal and low arterial blood pressure. J. Neurol. Neurosurg. Psychiat. 28, 449 - 452

35. Harrison, M.J.G., Thomas, D.J., Du Boulay, G.H.,Marshall, J. (1979) Multi-infarct dementia. J. Neurol. Sci.40, 97 - 103

36. Herrmann, H.-D., Dittmann, J. (1971) Steigerung des Glukose- Stoffwechsels von Kaninchen-Hirnschnitten durch Centrophenoxin. Arzneimittel-Forsch./Drug Res. 21, 984 - 985

37. Herrschaft, H.(1976) Gehirndurchblutung und Gehirnstoffwechsel. Meßverfahren, Physiologie, Pathophysiologie, Veränderungen bei den hirnorganischen Erkrankungen, Pharmakologie. Stuttgart; Thieme

38. Herrschaft, H., Gleim, F.,Duus,P.(1974)Die Wirkung von Centro- phenoxin auf die regionale Gehirndurchblutung bei Patienten mit zerebrovaskulärer Insuffizienz. Dtsch. med. Wschr. 99, 1707 - 1714

39. Herrschaft, H., Schmidt, H. (1973) Die quantitative Messung der örtlichen Hirndurchblutung in Allgemeinnarkose unter Normo-, Hypo- und Hyperkapnie. Anaesthesist 22, 442 - 456

40. Hoyer, S.: Der Aminosäurenstoffwechsel des normalen menschlichen Gehirns. (1970)Klin.Wschr. 48, 1239 - 1243
41. Hoyer, S.(1976) Hirndurchblutung und Hirnstoffwechsel im Verlauf eines organischen Psychosyndroms bei nichtbehandelten Patienten. In: S.Hoyer (Ed.): Hirnstoffwechsel und Hirndurchblutung. Amsterdam, Oxford; Excerpta Medica pp 1 - 8
42. Hoyer, S. (1978) Das organische Psychosyndrom. Überlegungen zur Hirndurchblutung, zum Hirnstoffwechsel und zur Therapie. Nervenarzt 49, 201 - 207
43. Hoyer, S. (1978) Blood flow and oxidative metabolism of the brain in different phases of dementia, in : R.Katzman, R.D.Terry, Katherine L.Bick (Eds.): Alzheimer's disease: Senile dementia and related disorders (Aging Vol.7). New York; Raven Press, pp 219 - 226
44. Hoyer, S.(in press)Gerontopsychopharmacological agents: Biochemical effects, in:G.V.R.Born, O.Eichler, A.Farah, H.Herken, A.D.Welch (Eds.): Handbook of experimental pharmacology. Psychotropic agents, part 2 (Ed.: F.Hoffmeister). Berlin, Heidelberg, New York.
45. Hoyer, S., Blaha, L., Erzigkeit, H., Weinhardt, F. (1978) Zusammenhänge zwischen Veränderungen der Hirndurchblutung und des Hirnstoffwechsels sowie psychometrischen Befunden bei Patienten mit einer Demenz. In H.Lauter (Ed.): Gerontopsychiatrie 6, pp 19 - 30. Janssen, Düsseldorf.
46. Hoyer, S., Hamer, J., Alberti, E., Stoeckel, H., Weinhard, F. (1974) The effect of stepwise arterial hypotension on blood flow and oxidative metabolism of the brain. Pflügers. Arch.351, 161 - 172
47. Hoyer, S., Krüger, G., Oesterreich, K., Weinhardt, F. (1976) Drug effects on cerebral circulation and oxydative brain metabolism in demented patients. 8.Int.Salzburg Conf.on cerebral vascular disease
48. Hoyer, S., Krüger, G., Weinhardt, F.(1978) Brain blood flow and metabolism in relation to psychiatric status in patients with organic brain syndromes. 9.Int.Salzburg Conf. on cerebral vascular disease
49. Hoyer, S., Oesterreich, K., Weinhardt, F., Krüger, G.(1975) Veränderungen von Durchblutung und oxydativem Stoffwechsel des Gehirns bei Patienten mit einer Demenz. J.Neurol. 210, 227 - 237
50. Hoyer, S., Quadbeck, H.(1978) Brain blood flow and metabolism in dementia. 11.C.I.N.P. Vienna
51. Jellinger, K.(1976) Neuropathological aspects of dementias resulting from abnormal blood and cerebrospinal fluid dynamics. Acta Neurol. Belg. 76, 83 - 102
52. Jones, J.V., Strandgaard, S., Mackenzie, E.T., Fitch, W., Lawrie, T.D.V., Harper, A.M.(1975) Autoregulation of cerebral blood flow in chronic hypertension. In: A.M.Harper, W.B.Jennett, J.D.Miller, J.O.Rowan (Eds.): Blood flow and metabolism in.the brain. Edinburgh, London, New York; Churchill Livingstone, pp 5.10 - 5.13
53. Kaasik, A.E., Nilsson, L., Siesjö, B.K.(1970) The effect of arterial hypotension upon the lactate, pyruvate and bicarbonate concentration of the brain tissue and cisternal CSF and upon the tissue concentrations of phosphocreatine and adenine nucleotides in anesthetized rats. Acta physiol. scand.78, 448 - 458

54. Katzman, R. (1976) The prevalance and malignancy of Alzheimer disease. Arch. Neurol. 33, 217 - 218
55. Kety, S.S., Schmidt, C.F. (1946) The effects of active and passive hyperventilation on cerebral blood flow, cerebral oxygen consumption, cardiac output and blood pressure of normal young men. J.clin.Invest.25, 107 - 119
56. Kety, S.S., Schmidt, C.F. (1948) The effects of altered arterial tensions of carbon dioxide and oxygen on cerebral blood flow and cerebral oxygen consumption of normal young men. J.clin.Invest.27, 484 - 492
57. Lassen, N.A. (1959) Cerebral blood flow and oxygen consumption in man. Physiol.Rev.39, 183 - 238
58. Lassen, N.A. (1974) Control of cerebral circulation in health and disease. Circulation Res. 34, 749 - 760
59. Lassen, N.A., Agnoli, A. (1972) The upper limit of autoregulation of cerebral blood flow on the pathogenesis of hypertensive encephalopathy. Scand.J.clin.Lab.Invest.30, 113 - 115
60. Lauter, H., Meyer, J.E.(1968) Clinical and nosological concepts of senile dementia, in: C.Müller, L.Ciompi (Eds.): Senile dementia. Bern; Huber, pp 13 - 27
61. Meyer, J.S., Gotoh, F., Tazaki, Y., Hamaguchi, K.,Ishikawa, S., Novailhat, F., Symon, L. (1962) Regional cerebral blood flow and metabolism in vivo. Effects of anoxia, hypoglycemia, ischemia, acidosis, alkalosis and alterations of blood p CO_2. Arch. Neurol.7, 560 - 581
62. Miller, J.D., Stanek, A., Langfitt, T.W. (1972)Concepts of cerebral perfusion pressure and vascular compression during intracranial hypertension. Progr. Brain Res.35, 411 - 432
63. Nemoto, E.M., Stezoski, S.W., Mac Murdo, D. (1978) Glucose transport across the rat blood - brain barrier during anesthesia. Anesthesiology 49, 170 - 176
64. Newton, R.D. (1948) The identity of Alzheimer's disease and senile dementia and their relationship to senility. Brit. J. Psychiatr. 94, 225 - 249
65. Nickel, J., Breyer, U., Claver, B., Quadbeck, G. (1963) Zur Wirkung von Aminoaethanol-Derivaten auf das Zentralnervensystem. Arzneimittel-Forsch./Drug.Res.13, 881 - 883
66. Oeriu, S., Winter, D., Dobre, V., Bruhis, S. (1973) Glucose transport across blood brain barrier as related to age and meclofenoxate treatment. J.Pharmacol.4, 497 - 503
67. Oldendorf, W.H.(1971) Brain uptake of radiolabelled amino acids, amines and hexoses after arterial injection. Amer.J.Physiol.221, 1629 - 1639
68. Oldendorf, W.H.(1976) Blood-brain barrier. In: H.E.Himwich (Ed.) Brain metabolism and cerebral disorders. New York; Spectrum Publications, pp 163 - 180
69. Olesen, J.: (1974) Cerebral blood flow. Methods for measurement, regulation, effects of drugs and changes in disease Acta neurol.scand.50, Suppl.57, 49-58
70. Pardridge, W.M., Oldendorf, W.H. (1977) Transport of metabolic substrates through the blood-brain barrier. J.Neurochem.28, 5 - 12
71. Patterson, J.L., Heyman, A., Battey, L.L., Ferguson, R.W.(1955) Threshold of response of the cerebral vessels of man to increase in blood carbon dioxide. J.clin.Invest.34, 1857 - 1864
72. Raichle, M.E., Posner, J.B., Plum, F. (1970) CBF during and after hyperventilation. Arch. Neurol. 23, 394 - 403

73. Rapela, C.E., Green, H.D. (1964) Autoregulation of canine cerebral blood flow. Circulat. Res. 15, Suppl.I, 205 - 211
74. Reivich, M. (1964) Arterial p CO_2 and cerebral hemodynamics Am.J.Physiol.206, 25 - 35
75. Rümmele, W. (1965) Die Behandlung der agitierten Zerebralsklerose. Dtsch. med. Wschr.90, 2118 - 2120
76. Sacks, W. (1976) Human brain metabolism in vivo. In: H.E.Himwich (Ed.): Brain metabolism and cerebral disorders. New York; Spectrum Publications, pp 89 - 127
77. Schmidt, H., Broicher, H. (1970) Klinische Erfahrungen bei der Behandlung von Zuständen zerebraler Insuffizienz mit Centrophenoxin (Hëlfergin). Med.Welt 21, 1432 - 1436
78. Severinghaus, J.W., Lassen, N.A. (1967) Step hypocapnia to separate arterial from tissue p CO_2 in the regulation of cerebral blood flow. Circulation Res.20, 272 - 278
79. Shapiro, W., Wassermann, A.J., Patterson, J.L. (1965) Human cerebrovascular response time to elevation of arterial carbon dioxide tension. Arch. Neurol. 13, 130 - 138
80. Shapiro, W., Wassermann, A.J., Patterson, J.L. (1966) Human cerebrovascular response to combined hypoxia and hypercapnia. Circulation Res.19, 903 - 910
81. Siesjö, B.K., Messeter, K. (1971) Factors determining intracellular pH. In: B.K.Siesjö, S.C.Sørensen (Eds.):Ion homeostasis of the brain. Copenhagen; Munksgaard, pp 244 - 262
82. Siesjö, B.K., Nilsson, L., Rokeach, M., Zwetnow, N.N. (1971) Energy metabolism of the brain at reduced cerebral perfusion pressures and in arterial hypoxaemia. In: J.B.Brierley and B.S.Meldrum (Eds.): Brain hypoxia. London; W.Heinemann Med.Book Ltd.,pp 79 - 93
83. Siesjö, B.K., Zwetnow, N.N. (1970) The effect of hypovolemic hypotension on extra- and intracellular acid-base parameters and energy metabolism in the rat brain. Acta physiol.scand.79, 114 - 124
84. Strandgaard, S., Mackenzie, E.T., Sengupta, D., Rowan, J.O., Lassen, N.A., Harper, A.M. (1974) Upper limit of autoregulation of cerebral blood flow in the baboon. Circulation Res.34, 435 - 440
85. Strandgaard, S., Olesen, J., Skinhøj, E., Lassen, N.A. (1973) Autoregulation of brain circulation in severe arterial hypertension. Brit. Med.J. 1, 507 - 510
86. Strandgaard, S., Sengupta, D., Mackenzie, E.T., Rowan, J.O., Olesen, J., Skinhøj, E., Lassen, N.A., Harper, A.M. (1975) The lower and upper limits for autoregulation of cerebral blood flow. In: T.W.Langfitt, L.C.McHenry,jr., M.Reivich, H.Wollman (Eds.): Cerebral circulation and metabolism. New York, Heidelberg, Berlin; Springer, pp 3 - 6
87. Terry, R.D. (1976) Dementia. A brief and selective review. Arch. Neurol. 33, 1 - 4
88. Terry, R.D. (1978) Aging, senile dementia and Alzheimer's disease. In: R.Katzman, R.D.Terry, Katherine L.Bick (Eds.):Alzheimer's disease: Senile dementia and related disorders (Aging Vol.7). New York; Raven Press, pp 11 - 14
89. Tomlinson, B.E., Blessed, G., Roth, M. (1970) Observations on the brains of demented old people. J.Neurol.Sci.11, 205 - 242
90. Wietek, H.F. (1963) Vigilität und Centrophenoxin. Arzneimittel-Forsch.13, 1102 - 1109

91.Wollman, H., Alexander, S.C., Cohen, P.J., Smith, T.C.,Chase,
   P.E., Van der Molen, R.A. (1965) Cerebral circulation during
   anesthesia and hyperventilation in man. Thiopenthal induction
   to nitrous oxide and d-tubocurarine. Anesthesiology 26,329-334
92.Wollman, H.,Smith, T.C., Stephen, G.W., Colton, E.T.,Gleaton,
   H.E., Alexander, S.C. (1968) Effects of extremes of respiratory
   and metabolic alkalosis on cerebral blood flow in man. J.appl.
   Physiol.24, 60 - 65
93.Wüllenweber, R., Gött, U., Szántó,J. (1967) Beobachtungen
   zur Regulation der Hirndurchblutung. Acta neurochir.16,
   137 - 153
94.Yoshida, K., Meyer, J.S., Sakamoto, K., Handa, J.(1966)Auto-
   regulation of cerebral blood flow. Electromagnetic flow measurements during acute hypertension in the monkey. Circulation
   Res.19, 726 - 738
95.Zirner, F., Wissel, M. (1966) Zur Anwendung von Helfergin
   (Centrophenoxin) in der Geriatrie. Med. Welt 14, 734 - 738
96.Zwetnow, N.N. (1970) The influence of an increased intracranial
   pressure on the lactate, pyruvate, bicarbonate, phosphocreatine,
   ATP, ADP and AMP concentrations of the cerebral cortex of dogs.
   Acta physiol.scand. 79, 158 - 166

Subject Index